LIVING

COURAGEOUSLY

POSITIVE

DR THULELAH BLESSING TAKANE

LIVING
COURAGEOUSLY
POSITIVE

INSPIRED
PUBLISHING

Living Courageously Positive
First Edition, First Impression 2020
ISBN 978-1-990961-47-2
Copyright © Thulelah Blessing Takane

Published by:
Inspired Publishing
PO Box 82058 I Southdale I 2135
Johannesburg , South Africa
Email: info@inspiredpublishing.co.za
www.inspiredpublishing.co.za

TABLE OF CONTENTS

DEDICATION

I dedicate this book:

To each family member and close friend that lost their lives to HIV. Had I known what I know now their lives would have been spared.

To family members, including mine who experienced the trauma of watching their loved ones die of HIV.

To family members and friends who were affected emotionally and physically while taking care of their loved ones.

To all my dear friends whose personal experiences of having to deal with HIV inspired the writing of this book.

To all my dear friends who have been affected directly and indirectly by HIV.

To all my dear family members and friends who have been my pillars of strength during this journey. I love you all from the bottom of my heart. May Daddy God water you as you have watered me.

To those who have been diagnosed with HIV and are about to discover healing, hope and restoration through this book.

ACKNOWLEDGEMENTS

I would like to give thanks, praise and honour to my Daddy God, my Creator, my Comforter and my Everything, the One who gave me a second chance to live and the one who has preserved my life until now so that I might tell of His grace and mercy to the world.

If mercy had not rewritten my life I would have fallen and died. I would also like to express my deepest gratitude to all my friends and family who have walked with me in this journey and to those who have given me platforms to share my journey.

INTRODUCTION

Hurting people, hurt others…
The writing of this book has mostly been motivated by the pain that I have suffered in my life because I have always sought complete healing for my heart. Sometimes it takes talking about your pain for you to heal. In order to deal with all of pain I have gone through I have found solace in writing. Thus, I decided to write this book primarily for the healing of my heart amongst other reasons.

It is important to note upfront that this book is written from the perspective of a born-again believer who believes in COMPLETE HEALING of EVERY SICKNESS AND DISEASE and who believes that the Word of God is alive and real. This book is thus written primarily from the perspective of sharing my experiences about waiting on the Lord through faith for His promise according to His Word that will never go back to Him empty.

Other reasons for writing this book are to reach:
Those who are infected with the Human Immunodeficiency Virus (HIV),
Those who are affected by the virus closely and those who are just interested in being educated about the virus.
Those who have been suffocating in the church and have felt that they cannot talk to anyone about their status because they will be judged or all they will hear is 'we will pray for you'.

Those who have been praying and waiting on the Lord for complete healing of either HIV or any other chronic disease.

Those who do not understand God and His ways yet.

People - especially new converts in the church - need to understand that we are not born 'born again'. I was only born again at the age of 22 and by that time I had embarked on sin like nobody's business. Making a decision to open my heart and receive Jesus Christ as my Lord and Saviour was the first step in a process of restoration of all that the devil had stolen from my life.

People need to understand that making a decision to receive Jesus as Lord and Saviour does not suddenly change things in your life. This is usually the first step into the process of becoming a new person and the focus is usually on the heart. If you had become pregnant out of wedlock, when you got born again the baby would not - all of sudden - melt in the stomach. You carry that baby until they are born and you walk through the process of being a new person in Christ and God gives you grace to take care of the baby. You also learn to take responsibility for your own actions and understand that there are consequences for every decision we make. If you had HIV, the virus remains in your body especially if you did not know and if you knew, and you happened to pray when you were born again, God could heal you completely, but He also might not, which means you might need to continue in your walk with God as a believer in His promises with the virus and trust Him in the process of your growth.

So when men and women, who are about to get married in the church, are asked to go for an HIV test if they have been sexually active before it's not that people are being mean or they don't have faith in God. It's because the reality is that anything could have happened and I have personally learned that HIV is a silent killer and the symptoms can take years to show.

In my journey of eight years since my diagnosis of HIV I have never had TB and skin problems. Instead I have always looked and felt very healthy - healthier than people who are HIV negative. Some symptoms might not even be attributed to the virus. A friend's mom went blind from HIV. She was quite elderly so they would have never thought that HIV was the reason. The only reason she decided to test is because my friend is a doctor and I think they were testing her blood for something else and then discovered that actually the blindness was a result of the virus.

As much as this book is about my journey of dealing with HIV, I saw it fit to share about my different life experiences in order to provide a broader context of how my life has played out to date and how grace has brought me through every season.

I have been inspired by others who have written their life stories and the powerful thing about writing is that it allows to re-visit your story over and over again because there are certain things a person picks up from a book at every moment they read it.

One day I was talking to a friend and as I was apologising about talking too much, this friend's response was 'Oh don't worry I actually love listening to you, you are such a story-teller'. That struck me and I realised at that it was time to start telling my stories in written form so that everyone who needs to hear them can access them and be healed.

I cannot remember how many times I have written and scrapped this book because of the emotions that came with the writing. At some point, I thought I had managed to write something, but I realised that every time I tried writing I was so full of anger towards myself and was covered with shame. When the right time came for me to start writing, I just flowed with emotions of gratitude. It eventually got to a place where I felt I had dealt with my hurt and anger issues by the grace of God. By having walked with the Holy Spirit in this journey I have learned so much about God, myself, people and life in general. I also understand that I am the light of the world. As the light of the world and the salt of the earth, there will always be opposition to what we have been destined to and sometimes not all challenges are from the devil, but that God allows them to happen for a specific purpose, like he did with Job. I have had a different perspective of the book of Job since my HIV journey, and so many times, I have felt like Job but - most importantly - I have come to understand why I have had to go through some experiences.

It is also important to admit that sometimes we suffer because of our own doings and God by His grace gives us strength to endure the consequences. As you read you will get to learn about my journey and how I came to make peace with some difficult situations in my life, especially the HIV diagnosis.

* Please note that the names mentioned in the book are not the real names of the people written about.

CHAPTER 1
IT'S POSITIVE

In 2012, on the 14th of July, these are the words that I heard which would change my life forever had I not had a relationship with God through Jesus Christ. I had decided to go for an HIV test. At this time I was at my peak when it comes to my health. My health had just become better over the years.

At the end of 2011 I was getting ready for my move from Cape Town to Johannesburg and - as per my custom - I fast at the beginning of every month. At that point of my life I had sense of transitioning into a new season and I wanted to focus on my relationship with God and on the new season I was about to embark on. I also felt that I did not want to make any relationship mistakes anymore. I had decided I did not want to be in a relationship with any man and so decided to spend most of December indoors fasting and praying.

On the 2nd of January, after breaking my fast I decided to take a walk to hire a movie. I later learned that this was probably a bad move - you will understand why I say this as you continue reading. After fasting a person needs to be very discerning as they are usually at their most vulnerable state. Their spirit is not only open to the heavenly realm but also to the demonic realm. Our example is Jesus (see Matthew 2:1-3):

Then Jesus was led up by the Spirit into the wilderness to be tempted by the devil. And when He had fasted forty days and forty nights, afterward He was hungry. Now when the tempter came to Him, he said, "If You are the Son of God, command that these stones become bread."

At the video shop I met a very handsome guy, I call him Max, who managed to sweep me off my feet although I tried very hard to run away from him. I really did try because I was determined about not entertaining any man at that point in my life. Max followed me around in the video shop and, after ignoring him, it seemed as if he had left me alone, only to find him waiting for me outside the video shop.

When I finally took a closer look, man oh man was he just gorgeous! His persistence attracted me to him even more. I have quite a strong character and I like a man who can stand up to me and Max was just that kind of man. He just would not back off. On the other hand, I felt this was my 'movie moment' right there. I used to love watching love stories and every time, when I had watched movies where a pretty girl was being harassed by a handsome man until he manages to get her attention and they live happily ever after, I would always wish I could experience that. Lo and behold my 'movie moment' was happening at the video shop. Be careful what you wish for.!

O but God is such a good Father who answers stupid prayers sometimes. I am reminded of another 'movie moment that took place in 2018 at Sandton City. I was with a friend of mine and I was assisting her shop for a convention that her organisation was holding. I was waiting for her while she went to the ladies room. A very handsome guy appeared in front of me and turned to look in my direction. Our eyes locked, he smiled, looked away and looked at me again and then turned and came to me. My heart was beating so fast and inside I was going: 'There goes my movie moment, there goes my movie moment'. He got to me, greeted me and I greeted back. My friend was out of the ladies at this moment and was standing next to me. This guy asked for my number. My friend started questioning who he was and why he was asking for my number. I gave him my number, but he never called. I think my friend scared him away. On a serious note, I believe the guy probably did not call because God was saving me from the unknown. You see, beauty does not come from the outside but from inside.

Going back to Max at the video shop, he finally got my attention and asked me out for a meal at that moment. I was completely charmed. We went to sit somewhere at a coffee shop. He bought me a muffin and coffee and he didn't eat. I discovered later that he's very healthy and doesn't just eat anything and to him muffins are 'junk'. I've always been very health, but this guy was just extreme and I loved that about him as it meant I would not have to force him to eat healthy.

We had a chat and then he invited me to his place to watch a movie and by that time I was head over heels so I agreed. He was so well mannered and he carried himself like a real gentleman. I even slept over at his place and 'nothing' happened. I had mentioned to him that I was born again and certain things were therefore forbidden - one of which is sex outside of marriage. At some point in our conversation, when I was asking about his stand in God, he told me he had been a believer before but was no longer practicing. I did not ask why. We continued to spend the following few days together without having sex. I discovered we had a quite a lot in common and I was so in love with him.

One day, things got heated and I let my guard down. After that day things changed. He became very distant until I moved to Johannesburg. When we met for the first time I had told him that I was moving to Joburg and I later discovered that he was also moving to Pretoria although he did not disclose this on that day. He finally moved to Pretoria and we connected again. I would not say we were in a relationship, as he only connected with me when it was convenient for him, but I was still so in love with him so I was excited when he did connect. There was no intimacy involved when we did meet face to face because I had made a decision to be celibate until I was married - as was always my resolution. All we did was just talk and argue a lot. I later discovered he was quite arrogant and rude which was very strange because my first encounter of him was the opposite. You could swear he was bipolar. It never made sense to me how he would be such a gentleman when we met and then turn into a very mean person at a later stage.

One day we were arguing because he had asked me to go to America with him, then played games and ended up going without me. He then said I should go for an HIV test. For some reason his suggestion kept on ringing in my head and on the 14th of June 2012 I went for the test. 'Til today I do not know why he suggested that I go for the test because when we were intimate at some point we had used protection. The last time I had tested for HIV was in 2004 and the results were negative. I do not know for sure if this was the case although, at that time, knowledge about the virus and testing was still fresh. Most health workers had no full knowledge of how the testing really worked, for example on the HIV test there could be a solid line and a faded line which could mean the test needs to be done again in order to confirm proper results. I learned about this when I had gone to test for the second time because the second line was faint and it meant I had tested positive.

Quite interestingly, it was the second time a man had asked me to go for an HIV test. The first man, Xolile, I had met in 2009 and he had just re-located from America and had been in exile there for many years. Xolile was pursuing me but at that time I was still on my journey of seeking God for my purpose. I had planned to always seek God and serve Him with my life. At the time I met Xolile, I was staying at a backpackers by faith and was just not in a good space in every way and in the most difficult wilderness season. I was very vulnerable.

I had met this man at a church where I was fellowshipping and because there were not many black people it was very easy for us to spot each other and connect. Initially I was not even attracted to him as I was really turned off by his 'slowness'. I remember he was trying to take my number and he acted as if he could not operate his cellphone. He was acting very dumb and strange, and while he was still pursuing me many times he would mention that we both needed to go test for HIV and I would ignore him. I started doing research on him and discovered that he was a very intelligent academic who had been divorced from his white American wife and had two children with her. I discovered all of this by Googling his name.

Google is the best thing that ever happened to us people. So when you meet with a man or woman, and you think you might be interested in them, Google them, do your research, please. When I confronted him he did not deny it. I finally managed to break away from him and continued to focus on God again. And I never went for the HIV test. It was the last thing on my mind.

So now back to 2012. Max asked me to go for an HIV test and I actually went. So here's the truth: At some point I was convinced that maybe Max had now made up his mind that he wanted to be in a committed relationship with me although at this stage, as far as I could see, he had not displayed any actions of wanting to be in a serious relationship. Every time we spoke we argued a lot as I found him, on many occasions, to be quite rude and arrogant and inconsiderate of my feelings. In spite of all of this I still had hopeful thoughts towards a possible lifetime relationship.

The other reason I decided to go for the test was that I felt that my faith in God was strong and if the results came back positive He would give me the grace to deal with it. As I have been growing older and maturing in God I have been developing bravery to confront things I had always been afraid of when I was not born again. Testing for HIV was braving up against what I was afraid of and I was ready to face it. At that time I had just enrolled for full-time doctoral studies with Wits as a fellow under the Wits Maths Connect Primary project. I have always felt that I would never pursue a PhD but here I was, having been given this opportunity based on the hard work I had displayed before. I felt the most courageous and nothing could get me down.

So when I went for the test at the Wits Clinic I remember sitting in front of the counsellor and having a conversation about the virus and her asking me, if the test came out positive, who would be the first person I would tell. I told her I was quite informed about the virus and have looked after friends who had been infected. I have close friends I would feel comfortable telling. So she pricked my finger and mixed my blood with the solution on the 'tester' then she closed it for a while. She then checked after a few minutes, looked at me with a sad face and disappointment in her voice, and said 'It's positive'. As she said that I had so much peace in me. I felt no different emotions at all. Then she said: 'What does this mean to you?' I said 'nothing' and told her that I trusted God would give me the grace to deal with it.

I shared my testimony with her of how God saved me from ectopic pregnancy when I could have died. I said I believe He is a God who heals. I told her that, in 2002, I suffered from ectopic pregnancy, which means I had fallen pregnant but the baby was growing in the fallopian tube and it exploded. I landed in hospital in a critical condition. It turned out that the fallopian tube had exploded 11 days before I was admitted because I had felt the explosion. It was a miracle I was still alive. On that day, I had a visitation from Jesus and He told me He was giving me a second chance at life. I gave my heart to Him and the following day I started preaching to other patients and three days later I was discharged and my life in Christ began.

I told the counsellor that my health had become better over the years and therefore I had no fears at all. In most cases, when a person responds positively or with faith, to such news, health workers think the person is in denial. To a certain extent, I do understand because there are people who go through a stage of denial but this is not always the case. Not everyone goes through the stage and I was certainly not the one. So, to conclude, the nurse told me that I needed to check my CD4[1] count whenever I was ready.

I told her I would come the following week. I left the Wits Clinic and went back to my office at Wits but still had no different emotions. Maybe the news had not sunk in yet. When I got to my office, I tried to do some work then reality finally hit me. I just broke down and cried. As I was crying, the Holy Spirit started reminding me of when God told me to change my diet in 2003. After I was born again I started learning

---

1 *A CD4 count is a test that measures how many CD4 cells you have in your blood. These cells are a type of white blood cell, called T-cells that move through your body to find and destroy bacteria, and other invading germs. HIV can destroy entire 'families' of CD4 cells and then the germs these cells find have easy access to your body. The resulting illnesses are called 'opportunistic infections – OIs' - because they take advantage of your body's lack of defence. A normal CD4 count is from 500 to 1400 cells per cubic millimetre of blood. (Source:* https://www.webmd.com/hiv-aids/cd4-count-what-does-it-mean#1)

about how God heals sickness and disease if you believe Him and so I started praying for healing for my minor sicknesses such as pains in my leg.

Time and again I would also suffer from bronchitis and sinus infections, and was on chronic medication, but God healed me. One day when I was praying Daddy (God) told me to change the way I eat and I did. Little did I know that my way of eating would preserve my health for the 10 years before my diagnosis. In fact when I back track carefully I started having symptoms in 2007 as I had intermittent skin irritations which affected my scalp and my face to the extent that the irritation was sometimes unbearable. I consulted doctors and dermatologists and no-one ever suggested that I do an HIV test. I guess no one would have suspected because, as I say, I was looking very healthy and fit back then and the symptoms I was experiencing were common for HIV. So whilst reflecting on this in my office, I immediately wiped off my tears and started praising God because it dawned on me how God had preserved my life. Talk about turning lemons into lemonade!

The following week, I went back to the clinic for my CD4 count blood test. One of the nurses drew blood from me, it was sent to the lab and then I had to go back for the results two days later. The nurse who was drawing bloods tried to counsel me by sharing a story of her brother who had been diagnosed with HIV but was now on [2]Antiretroviral treatment (ARVs) and was doing well. ARVs are NOT A CURE for HIV. ARVs keep the level (viral load) of HIV in your body low. When the viral load is low, your CD4 count is able to pick up and your immune system recovers and stays strong. When the viral load is 'undetectable' it means that the HIV virus cannot be passed on to someone else. Married couples, with one HIV+ partner, can plan to have children without infecting the other however they would need to

[?]   *ARV drugs work by inhibiting the various viral enzymes critical to the HIV replication cycle, specifically reverse transcriptase, integrase and protease, from which the ARV drug names are drawn. Source: https://www.google.com/search?sx-srf=ALeKk03xLqXVvc2L0wqoA4rzVJjo9RPQ1Q%3A1598457324134&ei=7IV GX97xB6HzxgPO_LqgBg&q=what+are+antiretroviral+drugs&oq=what+antiretroviral+drugs&gs_lcp=CgZwc3ktYWIQARgAMgYIABAHEB4yBggAEAcQHjIGCAAQBxAe-MgYIABAHEB4yBggAEAcQHjIGCAAQBxAeMgYIABAHEB4yBggAEAcQHjIGCAAQBx-AeMgYIABAHEB46BwgAELADEENQizBYjTNgwk1oAXAAeAGAAfIFiAGXEZIBBzMtN-C42LTGYAQCgAQGgAQdnd3Mtd2l6wAEB&sclient=psy-ab*

get all the necessary information from their doctor before proceeding with the process of having a baby. If the mother is the one carrying the virus the baby can also be protected from the transmission of the virus.

My experience is that most health workers who are not HIV positive themselves advocate for ARVs. I understand it is their job but I have learned that they need to give you more than just basic details about ARVs. One other important point that many people are not told is that a person's body can reject ARVs which means that either the body will not respond at all or the side effects can trigger other illnesses in the body. I personally had some of these experiences. I will give more details about this later in the book.

I then went back for the results and saw a different nurse. I remember this nurse looking at me very puzzled. She noticed that I was enrolled for a PhD and my CD4 count was 273, way below the normal count, but I was looking as healthy as ever. She started asking me how it was possible that I was looking so healthy with such a low CD4 count and the stressful load of a PhD. These instances always gave me opportunities to share my testimony of God's goodness and how He can preserve a life.

I started sharing my testimony of how I knew, without a doubt, that God had preserved my life because it was also not making sense to me. Instead of this nurse counselling me I was the one counselling her. She had also been studying and had shared how she was really struggling but by the time I left that room she was so encouraged. I always encourage people to get out of their pain sometimes and reach out to others because you will be so surprised that you thought your problem was a huge mountain only to find that someone else has a bigger mountain than yours. As much as I believe that my life has been eventful, I always meet people who I feel have more eventful lives in a more hurtful and painful way than mine. This always gives me reason to cheer up and be grateful to my Father God for my life.

The same year of my diagnosis, 2012, after discovering that my CD4 count was 273, I decided not to take ARVs as I still felt that healthy eating would sustain me but more than anything I was determined to trust God for complete healing. This decision was not based on

One of the most amazing experiences during this journey has been the divine leading of the Holy Spirit. There are decisions that I made which I know were inspired by the Holy Spirit.

any information that I had about ARVs and side effects, neither was it based on having information about specific foods that would help boost my immune system. It was solely based on the fact that my health had improved over the years and I was convinced that the way I was eating and my lifestyle of exercise would keep me healthy.

One of the most amazing experiences during this journey has been the divine leading of the Holy Spirit. There are decisions that I made which I know were inspired by the Holy Spirit. When it comes to making the decision about taking ARVs, one of the truths that people are not told, is that ARVs can be destructive to the liver besides the fact that they can also have very bad side effects. Therefore, if possible, people who test HIV positive need to delay taking ARVs until they really have to start taking them.

After receiving the news of my diagnosis I told my then Pastor as I wanted him to pray for me. Then I did something very interesting and shared with a group of ladies as a testimony of how God had preserved my life. I then shared at a women's conference, declared that God would heal me and that one day I would stand at the same conference testifying to my wholeness.

Sometimes I would wonder if I did the right thing by disclosing in all these instances but I now know that it was my way of declaring to the enemy that I was up for a fight. I also believe it was the beginning of breaking the silence about the stigma, especially in the church, as the Lord has revealed to me that many are suffocating from HIV and they don't know what to do as well as who to speak to because it is still seen as a big and incurable disease.

I continued to believe in God for complete healing and at some point I spoke to a gynaecologist who is a believer and who told me he does HIV management in his practice. During our conversation, I think we misunderstood each other as I had told him that I was trusting God for completing healing and therefore I wanted to be able to test time and again to see whether the virus was still in my body. I never wanted to be checking my CD4 count. He thought I had said I wanted to manage the HIV and I made an appointment for a consultation. When I got to his practice I was attended to by a very lovely nurse and she started talking about management and about doing a pap smear. I totally refused and told her I did not want to manage HIV as I believed that God had healed me. Where the pap smear was concerned, in hindsight now it could have been that I was really terrified as I was still in early stages of coming to terms with HIV. It was very awkward during the consultation and I'm sure they all thought I was crazy.

I continued praying and trusting God for complete healing. After being prayed for many times I tested again and again and the results still came out positive. During all those times I would be disappointed but I never lost faith in God. I still believed that one day He would heal me completely. I finally decided to not focus on the virus and I continued with my life as usual. I later went to Cape Town and reconnected with a friend - I call her Gladys. Gladys was one of the people who had made me aware of how counsellors of people with HIV can be affected by the experiences of other people and how they themselves can be depressed more than those infected.

I had met Gladys around the year 2001 while I was going about my business and was at a taxi rank. I cannot remember how we started up a conversation but she was looking very weary. I think I might have been coming from attending one of the workshops on HIV that had been conducted by health professionals at our church branch in Langa township in Cape Town and I think I must have happened to share with her where I was coming from. Our meeting was really by God's design. Gladys then started sharing with me that she had been working as a volunteer in counselling people diagnosed with HIV. She told me that she had been so weighed down by people's sad stories and she didn't know how to not carry other people's burdens. She told me that the situation was starting to affect her mental state.

I invited her to come to our church as I felt that it was - back then - full of people who were a real community that cared genuinely for each other. At that stage, our church had started being open and sensitive about HIV as we had people around us who had disclosed their status. Our services were always vibrant as the church was full of young black people. We would sing hymns, dance, and ululate. Sometimes myself, and three other friends, would offer up special items during our services.

Gladys started visiting our church and from then on we became very close friends. As time went by, I was born again and moved churches and places of work. Gladys was also born again at some stage and we continued connecting until she enrolled for a theology course. She was always interested in helping people and in finding ways to empower those in need. She was also someone who believed in education and empowerment. Every time I went to visit her she was always lively and excited about life and that always encouraged me. She always inspired me a lot to think about ways of making a difference in impoverished communities. At a later stage, when I left Cape Town, we lost touch. It was only after my diagnosis that we met again to catch up as I had travelled to Cape Town.

I told her about my status and how I had decided not to take ARVs. She was so happy that I had made that decision and advised me to not rush and take them as they have very bad side effects unless my immune system became really weak. I remember her exact words: "We will trust God for complete healing." Some people get offended when you say this to them. I have always been a crazy believer in miracles so I did not take offence at all. In fact, I was very encouraged that there was someone who shared my sentiments. My conversation with Gladys was so uplifting and I was so glad I had reconnected with her. She shared with me a story of someone who she knew and who the ARVs had really affected badly to the extent that sometimes it was as if this person was dying due to the side effects. The person Gladys told me about has written a book about her own HIV experiences and has confirmed what Gladys shared with me. She's a big advocate of ARVs in spite of her experiences and I respect that.

I continued living my life without ARVs but continued eating healthily, exercising and taking supplements. Although I was not sick, I struggled very badly with fatigue but I found ways of managing it by resting as much as I could and by taking energy boosters. Another thing that contributed greatly to my health is healthy friendships. I have become very close to my family members over the years and I have been deliberate in keeping friends who bring value into my life.

Being able to do the things that I love, and having people supporting me fully, has always played a big role in keeping my stress levels very low.

Being able to do the things that I love, and having people supporting me fully, has always played a big role in keeping my stress levels very low. Although I am a workaholic, I love what I do and I find it extremely fulfilling to be able to do work that makes a tangible difference in other people's lives. Getting feedback from some of the people I have helped, in some way over the years, has always given me reason to not give up on life and what God can do in and through my life.

66

---

*"It is bad enough that
people are dying of AIDS,
but no one should die of
ignorance"*

– Elizabeth Taylor

CHAPTER 2
EXPOSURE TO HIV

My first exposure to HIV was in 2002 through a friend who had disclosed her status to us, her friends. I'm going to call her Nobulumko because she's the bravest person I have ever known.

We were a group of very close friends at the time and I was probably much closer to her and knew more about her than anybody else. At that time the stigma surrounding HIV was still very rife, but one day she called all of us, her friends, and told us that she had been diagnosed with HIV. The one thing I will always appreciate about this group of people is that during this time we were so close and had each other's backs. Amongst us there was a lady who was much older and who was extremely loving, compassionate, approachable and peace-loving. Most of all she loved God with a passion and was serving Him and everyone wholeheartedly. She was such a role model to us who were younger. She also had a way of bringing us together whenever we had misunderstandings amongst us. We were truly blessed to have her as our 'mother'.

After Nobulumko disclosed about her HIV status, we all embraced her and assured her that we would be there for her no matter what. At that time she had been working as a waitress but after we heard the news an older friend of ours got her an office job. Myself and our older friend took Nobulumko in with us so that we could give her as much support as we could. She was also not comfortable about disclosing her status to her aunt who she had been staying with. Nobulumko had experienced a very tough life yet was very brave and strong. She was very smart, funny, diligent, very creative and loved to laugh. Her childhood was traumatic but she managed to come out of it and make something out of her life.

She started at her new job and by this time we were staying together. It was so normal staying with her - maybe it was because of the kind of relationship we had always had, of treating each other as sisters. We would still wear each other's clothes as we were almost the same size. She also loved and enjoyed cooking so she would cook most of the time. She had good reports about her new job and she was also going for counselling. At a later stage she said she wanted to move back to her aunt's place and was ready to disclose to her aunt.

We supported her decision as we had seen that she had been very strong and believed she was dealing very well with her status. She went back home and disclosed her HIV status to her aunt. Her aunt embraced her and assured her that she would support her in every way. Nobulumko's greatest fear had been that her aunt would respond negatively because

Her childhood was traumatic but she managed to come out of it and make something out of her life.

of the way she had always heard her talking about people who had been diagnosed with HIV, but she experienced the opposite. I later learned that it was not because her aunt was judgemental but it is human nature. I have also been in settings where people made ignorant comments about people diagnosed with HIV but until it hits home things change. Sometimes people don't even realise that they are being ignorant which is why it important for us to continue to educate people about how to respond with compassion at all times regardless of who has been affected.

Nobulumko then started going through a stage of depression and started believing that people could see through her that she had HIV. Sometimes we would watch TV and an advert on HIV would come up which would spoil her entire mood. She started withdrawing and showing signs of depression. When she went for counselling with our older friend she would not respond. She would give away all her money at the end of the month believing that she would be dying soon. Sometimes her aunt would call us at night and say Nobulumko was telling her that she needed to go to hospital because there were things moving up down her body. When we would get there she would refuse to go to hospital and say she was fine.

This went on for a few months. She even stopped coming to church and avoided being in our midst. We continued praying for her and supporting her as much as possible. Sometimes it would be hard on us because after she had given all her money away we would need to give her money to go to work and to buy necessities. We didn't really mind as we just wanted her to be well. It was so painful to all of us seeing our dear friend going through this.

After a while we decided to leave her alone until one day she came back and apologised for her behaviour and said she couldn't explain what was going on with her. She then told us that she was going to disclose her status at church on the 1st December the day of the commemoration of World Aids Day. Oh man she made all of us so proud. She stood there and told her story with so much bravery. Other people (who we would never would have thought were infected) also stood up to share their stories. It was the most emotional moment for all of us but the beautiful thing about that day is that everyone was embraced and many challenged about their attitudes towards people living with HIV.

After this event, some doctors and nurses in a separate branch of our church decided to conduct free workshops on HIV and availed themselves for counselling. I was one of the people that availed myself to attend these workshops and to offer counselling to anyone who was positive. I did not know about my status then. It has always been in my heart to reach out to people who are hurting and faced with difficult situations probably because I have been through a lot of trauma myself and therefore it makes it easy to relate with others.

During one of the workshops a lady who had been working as a counsellor at a clinic at UCT was giving a talk emphasising how laden with stigma HIV was and how everyone was scared of it including doctors, nurses and counsellors. She shared her own experience. One day she decided to do an HIV test. She said that when her results came back she looked at the paper and saw 'positive' and she fainted. While lying on the floor, she realised that she hadn't looked at the name of the person's results. Then she looked again and realised the results were for someone else. In these workshops the main message was that we need to be sensitive when it comes to the subject of HIV as it affects everyone, the same way as the coronavirus is affecting everyone now. These workshops empowered me a lot about HIV and made me sensitive towards people diagnosed with HIV.

My third experience was with a friend whom I had met at a ladies' gathering. I will call her Linda. Linda was a very pretty woman and very loving towards everyone. She loved to laugh. I was drawn to her and we became friends. Linda was born again and I was not, although I was committed at church and even teaching Sunday School. When I was born again I went to stay with Linda at her place and we attended Bible School together. We bonded so much as we both shared everything about our lives including failed relationships and disappointments.

One day she took me to visit her family members and one of her cousins was talking negatively about people who are HIV positive and I happened to be defending them. When we got back to her place Linda started opening up to me about her status. She told me she had contracted it from her first boyfriend who she has been faithful to. She said I was the second person who knew besides a male friend who had been very supportive. She said that when she had discovered her status she did a lot of research and realised she had to change her lifestyle as she had to buy expensive medication and supplements.

Linda also needed to consult with her doctor for regular check-ups. She had not opened up to me because she did not know how I would react.

Linda didn't know how much I knew about HIV but when she heard my response to her cousin she knew she could trust me. By the time Linda disclosed her status to me I was empowered enough to know how to respond so I embraced her and assured that I would support her in any way possible. We continued living together as if I did not know anything. Together we continued praying and trusting God for healing. It was hard especially for her because she really felt God was not answering her prayers. I continued to support and encourage her to not lose hope. At some point we parted ways as I moved to a different area because of work.

My fourth experience of HIV was with a friend and colleague who was also been infected. This was around 2007. We were working together for a non-profit organisation and one day she disclosed to me that she had been infected by her ex-husband and almost everyone around her knew her story. Sometimes we would go out for supper and when the time came for her to take her medication she would cause a scene and she would want us to leave immediately. She would run out of my car like a mad person, and she did this several times. It even became an excuse for her to exit every meeting and event.

I eventually removed myself from her as I could not understand her behaviour. I now understand how hard it was to deal with HIV back at that time because she had been given an instruction that she had to take the medication at a specific time and if she didn't something bad would happen to her system. So she was reacting out of fear that was probably inflicted upon her by others.

My fifth experience was with a friend's older sister who had been infected and was in denial for a very long time. I call this friend Mercy. Mercy gave up her life to look after her sister. I will always applaud Mercy for this gesture. I had watched her on many occasions being brave for her sister. Mercy was told by the doctor that her sister had HIV which had now become [1]AIDS (Acquired Immunodeficiency

---

1   *A disease of the immune system due to infection with HIV. HIV destroys the CD4 T lymphocytes (CD4 cells) of the immune system, leaving the body vulnerable to life-threatening infections and cancers. Source:https://aidsinfo.nih.gov/understanding-hiv-aids/glossary/3/acquired-immunodeficiency syndrome#:~:text=Acquired%20*

syndrome). Mercy's sister would not accept that she had HIV which meant they would never talk about it and about how she felt about the situation she was in. I think Mercy's sister really struggled with it. She was angry at the man who had infected her and was also angry at herself. I know, I've been there before, but I was fortunate to quickly stop being angry. I couldn't be angry at any specific person as I don't know who I contracted the virus from. However I was angry at myself for being careless. I was never angry at God because I have always believed in taking responsibility for my actions.

What made matters worse was that Mercy's sister had a daughter with this man. I would go visit them at Mercy's sister's home and at some point she was really ill but she always had a smile on her face. She would say "I'm going to be fine." She could not do anything for herself. She was in nappies and my friend was her nurse – God bless her heart. We would pray for God to heal her, but she eventually passed on. My friend later discovered that her sister had felt she had been a disgrace to her and her family hence she would never admit to their faces that she had HIV. She had felt ashamed and blamed herself till the end. Had

Immunodeficiency%20Syndrome%20Speaker,life%2Dthreatening%20infections%20 and%20cancers.

I was never angry at God because I have always believed in taking responsibility for my actions.

it not been for my relationship with God I probably would have felt the same shame my friend's sister felt.

My sixth experience was with a classmate I befriended when I was enrolled for a certain post-graduate qualification. She was married and had fallen pregnant, so she went for a check-up and in the process asked to be tested for HIV and she tested positive. She told me she knew that she definitely got it from her husband because she had been faithful in the marriage. When she asked him to go for a test. He refused and never wanted them to talk about HIV at all. I continued to support my friend until we graduated. They are both well.

My last experience was with a parent of a child I was teaching. The child was very problematic in class and I called her for a consultation and she came. Our relationship started then. The mother disclosed her status and some of her challenges. I supported her and also helped with handling the child as his behaviour was really stressing her out.

One day she had to be admitted to hospital as she had meningitis. I would go to the hospital, would pray for her and tell her that she needed to fight for her health because her children needed her. She finally recovered and was discharged from hospital. At the time she was admitted she had been staying with her boyfriend who was also HIV positive. They were not taking good care of their health so I started advising her on how to take care of herself. I then connected her with a work readiness programme. She later got a job, broke up with the boyfriend and looked after her children. She later met someone who she married.

"

---

*"Do not let the stigma
of fear and judgement
cripple you"*

– Thulelah Takane

CHAPTER 3
TRACKING THE SOURCE OF THE HIV VIRUS

HIV can be contracted through the following ways:

- Having unprotected sex with someone who has HIV
- Drug-users sharing needles
- From mother to child during pregnancy or breastfeeding
- Getting stuck with an HIV-contaminated needle
- Receiving HIV-infected blood transfusions
- Being bitten by a person with HIV
- Contact between broken skin, wounds or mucous membranes and HIV-infected blood or blood-contaminated body fluids
- Eating food that has been pre-chewed by a person with HIV

(Source: https://www.hiv.gov/hiv-basics/overview/about-hiv-and-aids/how-is-hiv-transmitted)

It's important for me to mention the possible ways of contracting HIV as people readily associate contracting HIV with having unprotected sex. I believe that if people were well educated about HIV there would not be so much stigma associated with the virus. The people who I knew had HIV knew they had contracted it through a specific person. While for many people it might help for them to know, I have found that knowing where it came from makes no difference except exacerbating hate for that person.

In some instances it could be that the person did not even know they had it because - believe it or not - HIV can be a silent killer. The truth is that I never dwelt on trying to think where I might have contracted the virus from because I really did not think it would make a difference. By the time I got the diagnosis I had experienced so much pain in relationships and I had learn to take responsibility for my own actions so that I could heal and move on with my life. Only one person has asked me where I got the virus from and I told them I didn't know and that's the truth. Some people have contracted the virus from an unfaithful partner in marriage and some have contracted it from birth.

It's really liberating to face the truth in life because it always sets you free. Facing the truth and confronting it in my life has helped me deal with many heartaches that could have ended in depression and bitterness. As much as I do not know how I contracted the virus I also cannot deny that I have engaged in unprotected sex with many different individuals.

When I was growing up I always dreamt of a relationship that would last forever. Naturally, I am person who is very committed and who gives her all in everything. So in all my relationships I was always looking for a commitment and I have always believed that commitment goes hand in hand with trust so I would trust my partners enough to have unprotected sex with them. I later realised that human beings are naturally selfish and in most cases always look out for what they can gain and before I was born again to a certain extent I was selfish. I got into relationships so that I could be loved and be happy and when I was not getting the love and the happiness I was looking for I would leave.

For many years I struggled with the fact that all my ex-boyfriends always wanted to sleep with me while I wanted to build a relationship. Whilst this was the case most of them did make me feel very special. I have experienced a lot of love and tender care in most of my relationships and because I did not want to lose that, I always gave in to having sex as I thought it would make them commit. In most cases though once they got what they wanted they left.

It always felt good to be told that I was beautiful and loved by my ex-boyfriends as I never experienced unconditional love growing up. My sister was always the pretty one who was loved by everyone and who was always told that she was beautiful. As for me, I grew up being told that I was ugly, had big teeth and looked like a small dog when I smiled. I was also called all sorts of names and was sometimes accused of doing things I did not do. So these men made me feel loved and in return it was easy to give myself to them without feeling like I was being used. There are a few relationship experiences that I would like to share in this book which I believe might liberate someone as they read.

In my first year at tertiary I had a boyfriend whom I had met at a party. He was a drunkard but was very handsome, sweet and kind when he was sober. We would do what boyfriends and girlfriends do as was the norm for young students, especially back then. He was studying Maritime Studies and their residence was at the Waterfront in Cape Town. Every weekend they would have parties at their residence and he would get so drunk that sometimes I would have to drag him to his room.

One day, he went to a party, drank and then came back and found me sleeping. He vomited on the floor. I was so annoyed and disturbed so when I woke up that morning I decided it was over between us. I left him sleeping. He tried to call me but I wouldn't come to take his call. So he did the craziest thing. He came to my residence and told the house mother that he was my brother and that he had brought news that our father had passed on. I wanted to strangle him but he managed to sweet talk me and we got back together. Then he graduated and went to work at sea and I did not want to be in a long-distance relationship so I broke up with him. We would still meet when he was in Cape Town when their ship was in South Africa and he always tried to get back together but by then I was already born again and was not interested in a relationship at all.

In the years 1999 to 2000, while I was doing my in-service training, I began a relationship with Sipho via email. One of those general emails had been sent by a colleague of mine and I targeted one of his friends who happened to have done some research about me. It turns out he also liked me although we had not met in person.

We communicated via email and phone calls for a while and then, one day, my colleague was going to do work close to this guy's place and I asked him to drop me off. I later discovered that he was an alcoholic and a womaniser, but was very lively, very smart and very loving. I had not known all this about him, obviously, when we first met. He was extremely cute, very cuddly and approachable and loved people. He would always cook for me and really spoil me yet we would go out almost every night and he would always drink and get drunk. He also smoked a lot and so spent a lot of his salary and credit card on alcohol and cigarettes. Unfortunately, his friends were just like him so nobody advised him to be more responsible.

When I started talking to him about his drinking problem, which was even affecting his financial status, he kept on promising me that he was going to stop but he never stopped. In addition to his alcohol problem he was a player and he was very good at hiding it because I did not know until we had broken up. One day I actually caught him red-handed but because I was so blinded by love for this guy it took me a long time to realise that he was actually cheating. We were both very adventurous and crazy and we spent a lot of time together so there was no way I could tell he was cheating.

One day, I decided to surprise him at work. He was working long shifts so his day shifts would end around 6pm. I decided that I was going to pass his work on my way to the Waterfront in Cape Town where I would wait for his shift to finish and then we would go home together. When I got to the security counter I asked for him and the security asked me if I was his girlfriend and I said yes. He took out a box of half-eaten pizza, a cooldrink and said my boyfriend had left it there for me. I was so dumb I didn't realise on the spot that that was kept for someone else as he did not know that I was coming.

I could not eat, nor sleep until I realised that I had to go for counselling on campus as I was still a student.

Then the security guard said my boyfriend had left a message that we would meet when his shift was over.

So I took the food and left. Then I came back to pick him up. I was still a little bit blind to what was really happening. I got to Sipho's workplace when his shift was over and waited for him by the security area. When he came down he was with a lady colleague who I knew and who also knew me as his girlfriend. This lady was apparently 'stranded' and needed us to walk her to the taxi rank. As we were accompanying her the mood was very awkward, and after dropping her off, Sipho started accusing me of being awkwardly quiet around the lady. The truth is I was just quiet as I still had not thought deeply about what was happening.

We fought that whole night and, of course, he was upset that I had messed up his plan of spending time with the lady. I decided to let the incident slide and we continued with our relationship. Then his previous girlfriend started harassing us and one day she came to his place, tore up my clothes and took some of them with her. It turned out that Sipho had never ended the relationship with this lady and was cheating on her with me. I know because he did the same with me.

I went home for the December holidays that year and, before I knew it, he had moved in with someone else who had become pregnant shortly after that. My heart was so sore. I was broken. I went to his place to beg him to take me back. All he told me was that there was nothing wrong with me and that the problem was with him. That week was the most horrible week of my life. I went into a deep depression. I could not eat, nor sleep until I realised that I had to go for counselling on campus as I was still a student. The counselling helped me a lot. I guess, because I desperately needed to get out of that depression, I made sure that I followed every word of advice that I was given by the counsellor.

During the counselling session, the counsellor asked me a few questions about my situation. I cannot remember all the details of our conversation but the one thing I remember is that she gave me a stick and a pillow and said to me: "This pillow is your boyfriend, I want you to beat him to death. I'm going to leave the two of you here and when I estimate that you are done I will come back." She left and I really beat that pillow, screaming my heart out. Then she came back and gave me a piece of paper. On it was written I am beautiful, I am loved, I am valued, I am worthy. She told me to put that piece of paper on my chest every day and say those words out loud. I did exactly as she had told me because I was so desperate to gain my life back.

I knew I wanted to live. In no time I was healed and I managed to move on with my life and totally forget about Sipho. I sometimes would bump into him and he would try to start a conversation but I would ignore him.

A while after breaking up with Sipho a lady who was one of his best friends confessed how she had been praying that I would break up with him as she knew that he was a player and that one day he would break my heart. She apologised that she could not warn me earlier and said it was tricky for her as they were really close and he would see it as a betrayal if she spoke to me. She also said she saw how much I loved this Sipho and that she thought I would not believe her and probably thought she was jealous of our relationship. I fully understood and was really grateful that she had shared that information with me. It gave me comfort to know that I had been saved from what could have ended up as being a huge disaster. At some point, Sipho had spoken to me about having a baby with me but I didn't take him seriously as I was still a student and I had always vowed that I would never have a baby unless I was married. I was so glad I never bought into the idea.

By the year 2000, in the last year of acquiring my National Diploma in Electrical Engineering, I was focused on my studies and decided to do away with all opposite sex relationships. However, I loved hanging out in night clubs and fun places just to destress, dance and socialise with people. One night an incident that shook me occurred. Myself and a friend were picked up by two guys to go to a nightclub. My friend claimed she knew the guys and I trusted her. She used to love having fun, drink a lot and was very flirtatious when she was drunk. I never used to drink. I have never drunk alcohol in my entire life and people always find it hard to believe me because of my extrovert nature. I have always hated alcohol because of the abuse my family suffered from drunkards when I was growing up. So when we were out in night clubs I would always make it my responsibility to look out for my friend although she was quite a tough cookie and a fighter.

One of the guys we went out with put a drug in my non-alcoholic drink which he had bought for me and – miraculously - the drug did not dissolve. I'm not sure if it was meant to but it came up through the straw as I was taking the first sip. I immediately realised that these guys were up to no good and our lives could have been in danger. I told my friend that we needed to work out a strategy to leave. After about 10 minutes my friend pretended to not be feeling well and asked the guy who had tried to drug me to take us home and he did. From that day on, I have never set foot in nightclubs again.

I realised that God was trying to talk to me and so I tried to give Him my attention. I started being more active at church and even started teaching Sunday School. I was not yet born again then but I was on the journey of searching for truth and purpose. Everything in my life was still driven by religion as I knew I had a deep desire to get to know God better and the purpose of my existence. I remember there was a time I was terrified of HIV. I couldn't even stand people mentioning it in my presence. I suppose it's because I knew the kind of lifestyle I had been living and the thought of having to test and discover that I was positive would just kill me on the spot. To a certain extent, these kinds of thoughts and my fears made me to open my heart to get to know God.

Whilst on this journey of discovering God and my purpose I got into a relationship with someone who was extremely sweet and such a gentleman. I call him 'Guy'. He was also a drunkard and a heavy smoker, and even smoked weed. Gosh, one could swear I had a magnet for these characters! In hindsight all these guys were extremely loving, caring and very gentle. I now realise that the bad habits were crutches in their lives which only Jesus can destroy because there are certain spirits that attach themselves onto a person and operate through them. My crutch was none of these toxins but promiscuity.

When Guy was sober we would have very long and meaningful conversations. He knew I was a committed church-goer and started sharing his past experiences with church and what made him drift away from God and the church. It was a very painful story. At this stage of my life, I was looking for a meaningful relationship in the same way I was looking for purpose for every area of my life. So I remained committed to church activities as these were a big deal to me. Initially, when Guy discovered that I was quite 'spiritual,' he tried to hide his habits until he couldn't anymore.

One Sunday morning Guy came to tell me that he was coming to church with me and he did. On the third Sunday, we had started 'The Alpha Course' and during our discussion time he re-committed his life to Jesus. From then on we decided to break up and just be friends. I was not born again yet but we spent a lot time talking about God and praying. Guy's life turned around in front of my eyes and then he started preaching to me and taught me the

Word of God while trying to convince me to fully commit to Jesus. Since the day he re-committed his life to Jesus he never touched alcohol, cigarettes or weed. I know because he was my neighbour and very close friend. God delivered him instantly. To me this was a miracle because I knew how indulgent he had been. I eventually was born again, and myself and Guy continued to be very good friends although I had moved somewhere else.

One day, he paid me a visit and we had a conversation about the importance of staying pure as children of God. He started by apologising for 'violating' me while he should have protected me. It was the first time I had experienced this kind of apology from a man. I also gave him an apology. I must say that it changed my perspective about men. It made me believe that there are men out there who are children of God, who are genuine and really kind. It made me believe that, one day, I would meet a husband just like him. Sometimes I wonder if he was meant to be the one but I just kept on pushing him away, especially when I was born again. He is married now and I know his wife is truly blessed.

When I was very young in the Lord, I was so serious about God that I wanted nothing to do with relationships. I am aware now that I did not mince my words about it and I came across as very aggressive to a lot of guys who tried to approach me. I remember there was a guy who was very cute and had a very cute smile who was trying to pursue me and I was very annoyed. This guy would call me just to check on how I was and I would get so hostile. One day, he asked me out for coffee and all hell broke loose! It was as if he had asked me to marry him. The guy eventually backed off.

At that stage of my life, I was so hungry for God and it seemed as if a relationship would be a distraction. I guess I had also just experienced relational traumas that made me closed up towards men. I only realised later that I had been hurting. Since I had moved and was staying very far away from church, I would spend my weekends at Guy's place so that I could attend church activities from Friday to Sunday then go back to my place. Initially, since myself and Guy were now friends we would sleep in the same bed, until he decided he couldn't anymore so he would sleep in the lounge when I was visiting him. The woman that got to marry Guy is truly blessed.

One weekend, I was visiting Guy but he was not home so I waited for him outside his flat. His flat was close to the entrance so everyone in their complex had to pass by his door to get to their flats. While I was waiting, Guy's neighbour 'Charmer' passed by and greeted me with so much charm. It was late afternoon. I was coming from the gym and was starting to feel cold. 'Charmer' asked me who I was waiting for and he noticed that I was getting cold. I told him I was waiting for Guy. He offered to let me wait for him at his place. He made me a cup of hot chocolate and we had a long chat as if we had known each other for years. Charmer had quite a sense

At that stage of my life, I was so hungry for God and it seemed as if a relationship would be a distraction.

of humour and so we laughed quite a lot while we were chatting. Right there we formed a bond and then he had to go and Guy was back. We exchanged numbers, he kissed me on the cheek and I was head over heels. From 'I don't want a man in my life' to 'I am so in love'. Sadly, it turned out that Charmer was also an alcoholic and a womaniser.

Truth be told, for the first time I felt like I had met my soul mate. I could not explain it. I have no doubt that he loved me genuinely. Based on the way he pursued me - even after chasing him away so many times and being there at the lowest times of my life - I'm convinced that maybe he also felt he had met his soul mate. But feelings can be misleading because here we are, still apart. By the time I had met him although I was not born again yet, I somehow knew that I should not be in an ungodly relationship. Guy, my previous boyfriend who had now become my friend, had been very influential and was very consistent in teaching me the ways of the Lord, so I knew some truths. But Charmer had just swept me off my feet and there was no turning back. I felt I could not let go of my soulmate so I was convinced. We connected in so many ways.

Our first date was at the beach. He was fun and we would both laugh so loudly at his jokes. I hadn't realised that I love to laugh until one of his friends started calling me 'Hlekayo' (the one who laughs). Charmer's behaviour and some events that started taking place started guiding me to suspect that Charmer was in a relationship and was staying with the person.

The truth later came out and I discovered that he had lied to me as he had said that he lived with friends. He had always avoided the idea of going to his place and always came to my place. I was fine with it initially but I later started seeing the signs. Believe me ladies, you can see the signs if you pay attention.

So I tried to break up with him because my principles had always been that I would not share a man. It was also giving me grounds to break up with the 'alcoholic'. I later discovered that the lady he had been staying with was pregnant, but they later broke up. I think she also got tired of his drinking and womanising habits. According to Charmer it was acceptable for a man to have multiple relationships and so he did not see anything wrong with what he was doing. I later realised that this had been a stronghold in his life since he had been born in a polygamous family. It became a struggle breaking up with him until one day I finally did.

Two weeks later I was admitted in hospital due to an ectopic pregnancy. I had fallen pregnant with his child but the child had been growing in my fallopian tube which had exploded. I had started being serious about church. How could I explain to my boss that her 'church' girl had fallen pregnant? I felt ashamed and initially had lied to my boss about the pregnancy until she spent more than three hours with me in hospital when I was not being attended to. She was planning to take me to another hospital so I told her the truth. She immediately asked for Charmer's number and told him to come. She knew we had broken up but she wanted to make it point that he was present since 'it was partly his fault' I was in this critical condition.

Charmer came and the first thing he asked me was what had I done to the baby. I suspect he thought I had aborted it. I'm so grateful that I didn't even have to consider such an option. This event became a turning point in my life as I met with Jesus face to face on my death bed on that day. One of the reasons why I would never turn my back on my relationship with God is that it did not take someone to convince me about salvation but Jesus revealed Himself to me and that will never change.

At some point, while still waiting to be attended to in casualty, I had a black out and it was during that moment when Jesus appeared to me and told me he was giving me a second chance at life, that He is my Lord and Saviour and I needed to live for Him. By the time I was discharged I had become a new person and my life changed completely. I changed churches, I changed my way of dressing, I removed my nose ring. It was important for me to take these steps as these were signs for myself that I was embarking on a new journey and people who knew me needed to know I had really changed.

66

---

*"HIV is not a death
sentence"*

– Thulelah Takane

CHAPTER 4

DEALING WITH LOSS, A SICK MOTHER AND MY OWN SICKNESS

I thank God that – naturally - I am a fighter but there have been moments in my life where I felt I had no strength to fight any more. In those moments, I usually surrender all to Daddy God. I have often wondered how people deal with pain when they don't have a relationship with God because there are situations that are just too much for a human being to bear. Sometimes, some of the situations we go through are just oppression from the devil and in those cases only God can intervene. I am always so grateful that I later got this revelation because - especially on my journey of dealing with HIV - I have needed God to intervene a lot of times, especially at times when I felt I was dying.

After my diagnosis in July 2012, I decided to remain strong and to focus on finishing my Masters degree. By this time I was so close to God that I knew His grace would get me through every step of difficulty. Then, in October of 2012, we lost my nephew who had been raised by my mother. It was a blow to the whole family. At this stage I had planned my life going forward around my nephew as I was planning to take him through varsity. I had already applied for him to study at Rosebank College. His passing meant I had to reschedule my life. Not only was this painful but losing him was the most traumatic. But then again my natural strong character had to kick in for everyone else.

My mother was the most affected. Why her? Why had God forsaken her? She had lost a son before and this one had come as her comfort but now he was also gone. She then got diagnosed with a heart failure at the beginning of 2013 and was in and out of hospital that whole year as well as the following year. This was until we decided to put her on medical aid and have her admitted at a private hospital. During the illness of my mother, there were times when my own health was weak and I would hide from my family members as I still had not disclosed my HIV status and I did not want them to have to worry about me too. After getting my mom admitted at a private hospital she was diagnosed properly and received the correct medication to stabilise her heart. She started to become better but it meant I had to re-shuffle my priorities. I had to find financial stability so that I could assist in supporting her. All of these experiences affected my PhD progress. Between myself and my sisters we had to make her our focus and also be strong on her behalf.

In 2017, my mother went for her yearly check-up for her heart. The doctor was quite surprised that my mother was still alive and functioning well because the x-ray showed that her heart was perforated and was not in a good state. This news did not worry us as my mom had been in better health than before. The only thing that apparently had been bothering my mom, which she told the doctor about, was that she had a constant sense of discomfort in her chest and the doctor suggested that she was admitted so that she could be examined.

When they did the examination they discovered that she had lung cancer. We were then directed to an oncologist to see how far the cancer had spread. We discovered it had spread to other parts of the body and was at stage 4. The oncologist told us about the possibility of chemotherapy but also made it very clear that it did not guarantee that the cancer would go away. She also said it would be more painful since they would have to operate on Mom and implant a port through which they would insert the chemo treatment. My Mom said she wanted to go back to the Eastern Cape and think about it.

Towards the end of 2017 we took her back from the Eastern Cape and she stayed with my sister. We just witnessed her waste away. In December of 2017 she was really not well and my sister was heavily pregnant. She had been given strict instructions by her doctor to not move around as she was close to giving birth. So I had to be the one running around on both their behalf. The best thing a person can live for is to be able to be there for their loved ones. Again God gave me the most supernatural strength to be able to run around and serve them.

The other blessing that we were praying for, since my mom had lost two sons, is that my sister would give birth to a son. God heard our prayers as she lived to see my nephew arrive in the world although by this time she had already given up on life and was ready to exit the world. We continued to trust God for her healing. We did all we could, from prayer to getting her the best treatments, but in May 2018 she finally passed on after having been in hospital for a month.

When she had been admitted my sister had just given birth and her baby was just over two months old. I had just started at a new job and my sister called me in the early hours of the morning just as I was preparing to go to work. I got to my sister's place and the ambulance came to take her. For some reason the hospital where we would usually take her was full and she was taken to a different hospital which turned out to be a blessing in disguise because the doctor who attended to her was both a physician and an oncologist, which we had struggled with at the other hospital. When my mom was getting ready to be admitted they put a drip in her and she cried like a baby from the pain. I will never forget that moment. My heart was so sore seeing her in that state, but again I had to hold my tears and be strong for her.

Then a very sweet young doctor came to attend to her. He was so gentle to her and even allowed me to be present while he was working on her. He made her feel so comfortable. Another nurse came to talk to me, also with so much kindness, and just encouraged me. I think she could see the seriousness of the situation. I was in hospital that whole day until she was properly settled in a ward. That whole month I had to wake up at 3am, get to work at

I have needed God to intervene a lot of times, especially at times when I felt I was dying.

5am, work until 3pm. Leave for the hospital to go and attend to my mom as she was refusing to eat and was sometimes rude to the nurses. I would leave the hospital around 5pm, get home and do some more work. That month I saw the hand of God yet again. I cannot explain the kind of strength I had to run around like I did that month. Yet again, I am so grateful to Daddy God that I had such an opportunity to serve my mom and my family at the time when they needed me the most.

The hospital became my second home and some of the nurses, as difficult as my mom was, went out of their way to make my mom as comfortable as possible. The day before my mom passed on it was Mother's Day. Myself and my sisters went to visit her at hospital and we celebrated with her and even took photos. The following day, which was a Monday, she slept forever. I had to be the one to go home to the Eastern Cape to start preparing for the funeral, again there was more running around there, but God! He sent me angels from all over who made my burden light and I had people from my church, colleagues and friends calling and depositing money. I will forever be grateful.

I'm sure you are wondering why I am sharing all of this while this book is meant to be about my journey with HIV. You see, what you need to understand is that HIV does not like stress. Stress makes your immune system weak, and your health deteriorates quite quickly. Everything I have spoken about was stressful but instead of my health deteriorating it became better and better. One of my greatest weapons has been Prayer. I love to pray and to intercede and so I have always found strength in communicating with God and in taking back whatever the enemy has stolen from me through Prayer. When I got the revelation of what prayer can do I made it a point that I would make it my every moment's priority. 1 Thessalonians 5:17 says "pray without ceasing", which means PRAY ALL THE TIME. During that month when my mother was in hospital I would pray for an hour before making my way to work. Sometimes I would fast and then pray in my car during lunch time. My mom's funeral proceedings went so smooth with so much unity between myself and my sisters as well as so much peace with the entire family.

When I got back to Joburg after the funeral people were so amazed at how strong I was. I was not trying to be strong. I was strong. God had given me an opportunity to serve my mother while she was still alive. She was born again and loved and had served God in her own way. She had been in pain for years and was ready to rest. That month, God prepared our hearts for her departure and we had an opportunity to say goodbye on Mother's Day. What more could we ask for? For me, the chapter was closed as I was comforted.

"

---

*"I shall not die, but live,
to declare the works of
the Lord"*

– Psalm 118:17 NKJV

CHAPTER 5
FACING THE GIANTS

I call this chapter 'facing the giants' because there are things that pose as giants in our lives that sometimes seem so big they seem impossible to overcome. In this chapter, I share my experiences of giants I had to confront at some point in my life.

In 2013 during the month of September, I attended a women's church conference and a lady gynaecologist - who I knew and was quite close to - was one of the guest speakers. Her talk was focused on advising women about the importance of taking care of their health by making sure they do regular check-ups and stay informed about health issues that usually affect women. Another lady Pastor shared a testimony of how God had healed her and her husband of sicknesses they had been diagnosed with. As these women started sharing, the Holy Spirit started ministering to me and I was just weeping the whole time. I have always thought I had it together when it comes to health issues - after all I was in good health and relatively strong although I was struggling with fatigue. The reality is that during these women's talks at the conference, when suggestions about having a pap smear were made, I started imagining the possibility of being diagnosed with cervical cancer and terror took hold of me. In my mind I was thinking: 'Please Lord, I cannot handle another chronic diagnosis. HIV was just enough for me.'

I don't know why my mind went to the worst. I suppose that when you have gone through a lot of pain you tend to develop paranoia. I later discovered that these were lies from the enemy. I also later discovered that when you are going through pain you focus so much on the pain and are vulnerable to the extent of losing consistency of praying and speaking the Word into your situations. You then start to entertain the voice of the enemy that says: 'You are going to die', 'You've been praying for many years now, God is not going to heal you, He has forgotten about you, He is punishing you for your sins'.

Another thought that was going on in my mind was that I was so fed up with being poked by doctors. I felt like all my life I had been a sick case and had been in and out of doctors' rooms. From when I was small I had struggled with hay fever and I was on chronic medication for years until God healed me and I came off the chronic medication. This part of my life, where I was a "doctor's case" was just too much for me. Now that I was a child of God I had learned that our faith would result in abundant life and so I chose to just believe God for healing of my ailments - even HIV. I became tired of being convinced that I could live with HIV and be healthy. I had refused to 'manage' it.

After the conference I made an appointment to meet with the guest speaker lady gynae. Fortunately, she agreed to meet for coffee. When we met, I shared my story and my fears. She spoke to me with such gentleness as if the Holy Spirit himself was talking to me. She encouraged me to do the necessary tests which involved a pap smear and also encouraged me to not shy away from taking ARVs should my CD4 count become too low. One of the things she explained to me - which I believe most women need to know - is the importance of doing a pap smear every year. If cancer cells are discovered within

Now that I was a child of God I had learned that our faith would result in abundant life and so I chose to just believe God for healing of my ailments

three years they can be fought without rigorous treatment unlike if it is not known when the cells had started developing. During my conversation with this lady I felt such a gentle comfort and assurance from the Holy Spirit that all was well and that I did not need to be afraid as Daddy God had my back. Now I had the courage to face my giants and I felt peace in my spirit to do as per the doctor's counsel.

The following week I went back to the Wits Clinic to do another CD4 count test. This time it had gone down from 270 to 163. (Remember a normal person's CD4 count is between 500 and 1500.) What was a surprise to the nurse who I was consulting with was that I was as healthy as a horse and I was looking healthy too. I knew the grace of God was keeping me. But at this stage I was ready to start taking ARVs as I was battling with fatigue. The nurse then advised me to find a doctor. She explained to me that before taking the ARVs I would need to do all the necessary tests such as TB, liver, kidney, etc., to establish that there were no infections. She also explained that since I was on a medical aid the doctor could fill in an application to put me on a chronic programme so that the medical aid could cover the ARVs and the management of the virus.

I had to find a doctor who was within the cover's network and was very fortunate to find a very nice lady doctor who became a close friend. We did all the tests, including a pap smear, and all the results came out clear. I was so relieved, you have no idea. Truth be told, I was so terrified and was praying very hard that none of my organs were affected, especially my liver. What I got to discover later on is that the liver and kidneys are the most important organs in the body so if they are not functioning well, the body could suffer complications and more so it is not be possible to take the ARVs until these recover.

Once we had established that my organs were operating perfectly, the doctor put in an application for the medical aid to put me on a chronic programme and it was successful. I started taking TRIBUSS from the beginning of 2014. I remember doing research on the Internet about side effects and this is what I found:

- Appetite loss
- Lipodystrophy (a condition that causes people to lose or gain fat in certain body areas. This may make some people feel self-conscious or anxious)
- Diarrhoea
- Fatigue
- Higher than normal levels of cholesterol and triglycerides
- Mood changes, depression and anxiety
- Nausea and Vomiting
- Rash
- Trouble sleeping
- Dizziness

(Source: https://www.healthline.com/health/hiv-aids/antiretroviral-drugs-side-effects-adherence)

The side effects that I would say I had were dizziness, loss of appetite and fatigue. I escaped the others because I'm generally an active person and I exercise regularly. I also escaped vomiting because I am not a person who gets easily nauseated and I have been fortunate in that I have never vomited in my life. The one side effect that affected me really badly was dizziness and constant headaches. These went on for the whole year of 2014 and were very bad. I lost a lot of weight to an extent that I would get extremely cold even in summer.

One of my friends, who did not know about my health challenge, would make fun of me about always being covered even in summer and I would just laugh and brush her off. I never used to take offense as she did not know what I was going through. The ARVs destroyed the fat in my body so that my bones started being exposed and if I bumped into something it would feel like I have been hit by a metal object. I also could not kneel as it would feel like my bones were touching the floor. At one point, the headaches were so severe that I thought I was dying so I went to see my doctor. She examined me and told me that there was nothing wrong with me and that I had to endure the side effects until they subsided.

I was so sickly and was experiencing a lot of discomfort. It was strange because before I started taking the ARVs my health was perfect but now I was so sick and uncomfortable.

"

"And when I passed by you in your
blood and saw you struggling in
your own blood, I said to you in
your blood, 'Live!' yes, I said to
you in your blood, 'Live!'

– *Ezekiel 16:6 NKJV*

CHAPTER 6
A BREAK THAT GAVE ME A 'BREAK'

Whilst trying to come to terms with the side effects from the ARVs I tried to focus my energies on my PhD and project work. One day I got a call from my supervisor as she had noticed that I was not well. I broke down while I was speaking to her on the phone. She came to see me and I told her what was going on. She suggested that I take time off the project and she motivated for me to get an extension for my PhD proposal. This break made a huge difference. The side effects continued to affect me to the extent that it would become difficult to wake up in the morning. I would snooze my alarm from 6am to 9am with my body refusing to wake up. I was forced to wake up in the mornings so that I could eat and then take my supplements in order to rebuild my immune system.

One morning I was lying on my bed feeling so sick and alone. I just couldn't take the discomfort anymore as most of the time it really felt like I was dying. Thoughts were going on in my mind that I am always there for everyone. I always go out of my way to reach out but there I was, alone with no one reaching out to me. As much as I needed to reach out to people I felt that people should know that I am not well because I am always deliberate about checking on others and in the process finding out if they are not well.

I was having my pity party with Daddy God and whilst I was at it I received a call from a friend to who I had disclosed my HIV status. The only reason I had told her was because she had been very sickly and was feeling so down and - as a way of encouraging her - I shared my story with her more as a testimony of how God had preserved my life. Initially she did not believe me because I was looking very healthy and she had always known me as someone who is always courageous and full of faith. When she called, she asked where I was and said she had taken time off work so that she could come and cook for me and spend the day with me. Look at God! Indeed he is attentive to the prayers of his children as He says in Psalm 34:15

"The eyes of the Lord are on the righteous, and his ears are attentive to their cry" (NIV)

On the day my friend came I had an awakening that there are people who want to be there for me but I need to reach out. I also realised that I always portray myself as someone who has it all together, maybe without realising it, because my nature is generally jolly and bubbly, so people would never think that maybe I am not fine. So I have since learned to reach out but I also have a lot of close friends and family who are deliberate about checking on me and it blesses my heart. In life we all need to feel loved and appreciated as it makes it easy to carry our heavy burdens that life always throws at us.

In the midst of everything I was going through I made a commitment to God that my condition would not affect my service to Him. My faith in God became stronger as it became apparent that He is the only One that could carry me through this journey. I even made a vow that I would continue serving Him through music ministry and I would rather drop dead in the presence and service of my beloved Father. I have found that it is important to pause when one is faced with some kind of a tragedy and examine one's relationship with God to hear what He is saying and to understand what God is doing in

"The eyes of the Lord are on the righteous, and his ears are attentive to their cry" Psalm 34:15

a certain season. I am so amazed at how Daddy God always gave me an understanding of every season in my life although it would sometimes be painful. I would always find peace in knowing that all things would work for my good (Romans 8:28) and that He would not leave me or forsake me as per His promise in Hebrews 13:5-6:

"Let your conduct be without covetousness; be content with such things as you have. For He Himself has said, " I will never leave you nor forsake you." So we may boldly say: 'The Lord is my helper; I will not fear. What can man do to me?'

I used the break that I was given by my supervisor to reconnect with myself, to seek God more and to fight to stay alive by claiming my life back from the enemy. Around June in 2014 I was feeling so much better and I had started with writing my PhD proposal again. I managed to attend Research School where I got ideas that helped me to wrap up by the end of June and I submitted my proposal for examination. It came back with no corrections at all, thanks to my thorough supervisor.

“

---

*“With long life I will satisfy him,
and show him my salvation”*

– *Psalm 91:16 NKJV*

CHAPTER 7
DECIDING TO STOP TAKING ARVS

I need to make a disclaimer before I tell my full story of why I stopped taking ARVs. I believe in science and doctors. I believe that science is not separate from God, but I also believe in miracles where science falls short. I believe that we all have different journeys and some people put their faith in God while taking medication and others make choices to have faith in God solely.

I believe people's choices and beliefs should be respected as we all have different experiences, some of which can be so painful that we might feel the need to make decisions that are contrary to the norm. I have been condemned so many times for making this decision but it has also given me the opportunity to help people get out of their own ignorance. So I would not be surprised if you are also condemning me as you read, but I suggest that you read to the end so that you can understand why I made the decision.

My challenge to many people is that if you have never done an HIV test, please keep your comments to yourself because if you were in the same boat you would make the same 'stupid' decisions. Many people do not know their HIV status yet they are the first to make comments about how people with

HIV should live. It's being judgemental about an experience a person has no idea about. If you have never experienced what it's like to feel like you are dying from the side effects experienced from ARVs then I suggest that you rather keep your comments to yourself. I have learned to rather pray for people who carelessly say things they know nothing about and, like Jesus on the cross, I just say 'Father forgive them for they know not what they are doing'. When you have suffered pain in the journey of battling with HIV, it gets to a point where no human being can get to you. You also learn to develop a thick skin otherwise you will end up being depressed by people who are ignorant.

Towards the end of 2014 I was extremely sick from the ARVs. In addition to weight loss, loss of appetite, and always feeling cold I started developing unending chest pains and coughing. I consulted with my doctor many times and she could not find anything wrong, but kept on giving me cough mixtures that would get finished but with no recovery. I then went to see a doctor in Cape Town who specialises in natural medicine and he discouraged me from eating fruit and said they were over-working my liver. He prescribed his natural supplements which I tried but still did not get better. I felt like the woman with the issue of blood who had spent so much money going from one doctor to another seeking for help, until she met with Jesus…

Just then a woman who had suffered for twelve years with constant bleeding came up behind him. She touched the fringe of his robe, for she thought, "If I can just touch his robe, I will be healed." Jesus turned around, and when he saw her he said, "Daughter, be encouraged! Your faith has made you well." And the woman was healed at that moment (Matthew 9:20-22 NLT)

I could not get myself to stop fruit as these were pretty much what I was eating, and I had discovered from research and personal experience, that I had survived the virus for so many years because of the raw foods including fruit that I was eating. Besides I really love fruit!

My health continued to deteriorate to such an extent that one day I had a conviction and peace in my heart about stopping the ARVs. I decided that the Word of God would be my medicine. Every day, when I woke up, I started mediating on the following scriptures and I would say them out loud. I still do:

"My son, give attention to my words; Incline your ear to my sayings. Do not let them depart from your eyes; Keep them in the midst of your heart; For they are life to those who find them, and health to all their flesh." (Proverbs 4:20-22 NKJV)

"Do not be wise in your own eyes, fear the Lord and shun evil. This will bring health to your body and nourishment to your bones." (Proverbs 3: 7-8 NKJV)

"But he was pierced for our transgressions, he was crushed for our iniquities; the punishment that brought us peace was on him, and by his wounds we are healed." (Isaiah 53: 5 NIV)

Before I knew it all the illnesses that I had developed, owing to the side effects of the ARVs, stopped and my health went back to normal. I continued speaking the Word, eating healthily, taking supplements and exercising. I still continued to battle with fatigue but God would give me grace to manage it and I would still be productive. I then went to test again and the results still came back positive. I must be honest and say that every time the results would come back positive I would be very disappointed but I would brush the disappointment off and continue with my life and trusting God. I would remember my allegiance to Him that I would give Him worship and serve Him no matter what because I got to understand that my body is infected with HIV but not my soul and if it happened that I died my soul would be saved and the HIV would go back to dust with my body. I continue to rest in that knowledge. I really wish God's children would get knowledge from the Word of the God so that they would not perish (Hosea 4:6).

During my journey with HIV, I felt so much freedom not because I was without pain but I really experienced what God means when He says in His Word that *'... If you hold on to my teaching, you are really my disciples. Then you will know the truth, and the truth will set you free" (John 8:31-32 NIV)*. You know there are people I listen to that fascinate me by how they narrate their lives having turned out as planned since I am a great planner and organiser and there are some areas of my life that have played out as planned, but the truth is that my HIV journey is one I had never imagined. So, in instances like these one cannot help but rely on the leading of the Holy Spirit.

The beautiful thing with having an intimate relationship with God is that He leads you in ways you would have never imagined. There are many decisions that I made that I know it was purely the leading of the Holy Spirit to the extent that sometimes, when people ask me how I went about doing certain things, I cannot explain my reasoning in a way that really makes sense. For example, how the Holy Spirit led me to start taking certain supplements and eating certain foods without needing to research what they would do to my body. I would later discover that they would be boosting organs that would be really problematic if they became deficient from the virus. I would later discover some of this information just by the way, sometimes from listening to health practitioners and specialists.

From the beginning of 2015 until 2017 my health was perfect with no discomfort at all. Then I started having gum infections and bad pain in my gums. I would experience bleeding when brushing my teeth. I consulted with a dentist. Although I had not hidden my HIV status I had not disclosed that I was not on medication. The honest truth is that, at some point, I was so oblivious to the virus that I was not associating any of my discomfort with it. According to me I was healed and was just waiting for the manifestation.

The dentist suggested that I brush my teeth regularly and also use a mouth wash. The truth is this should be our daily routine anyway. Then I started having back pain and I went to consult a physiotherapist. She associated the back pain with sitting for long hours writing as well as with bad posture. She suggested that I become more active and do exercises after about an hour of sitting. Fortunately for me, exercising has always been my thing from a very young age so I took her advice and became deliberate about exercise even if it was for a short time. Because of fatigue from my weak immune system I could not exercise for more than an hour. I could not even run anymore nor walk for long without taking breaks in between.

I then started having pain in my left leg, especially when exercising. At this stage I had a personal trainer who suggested that I buy new trainers and also consult with a physiotherapist. He helped me buy new trainers and I went to see the physiotherapist who did not tell me anything that I did not know. I always consulted just to make sure that nothing was going seriously wrong with my organs. I also started experiencing excruciating abdominal pains. These pains were strange because they would come and go and I would feel them mostly at night before I went to bed. They would be so bad that sometimes pain killers would not work so I would lay my hands on my abdomen and I would pray, speak the word over my body and command the pain to go. The pain would really subside and then I would sleep. I later discovered that the pain was caused by fizzy drinks and grape juice. I'm not really into fizzy drinks that is why it took so long to discover the cause. When I do drink them I usually drink Appletiser or Grapetiser on special occasions. I then started eliminating them from my diet and I never got the pain again. I also started taking calcium and magnesium supplements to strengthen my bones and I continued to exercise.

From 2017 to 2018 I had a very stressful job. My stomach started feeling bloated so badly that one day I could not walk because of the pain so I had to go see a doctor. As I entered the doctor's rooms this tiny black woman who was locuming at this practice received me and immediately I decided to not even entertain negative thoughts that 'she is so young what does she know'. So I had my urine tested and brought it to her. Before we even started discussing what was wrong with me she received me with so much warmth and professionalism. I was also admiring her as she was also very pretty and had dressed very smartly.

She then looked at the results of my urine and exclaimed that the results showed that I was as healthy as a horse. Remember I mentioned that I had a stressful job? Under normal circumstances, because of my condition, I should avoid stress because this could affect my immune system badly. But here I was getting this good news. Every time in my life that I felt like there was a flood coming against me God would always show up in small ways to encourage me and this was one of those moments.

This tiny gorgeous doctor then asked me what was my secret for keeping so healthy. I told her I eat healthy, I exercise and I take supplements and I really try to stay encouraged as much as possible. Then she asked if I take probiotics and I said no. She then suggested that I started taking them and then began taking me through a lecture of what happens in the digestive tract when a person takes tablets and what the role of probiotics then becomes. She was even drawing pictures for me. I was so impressed with this lady and I felt so encouraged.

During our conversation she started sharing that she was not really a GP but a dermatologist, however her practice had burnt down. She went to say: 'I don't let anything get me down in life'. So here I am feeling as if the world is falling on top of me - with a chronic disease, a stressful job and bloating - and God sends an angel to tell me life is not all that gloomy! I left that practice feeling so on top of the world. I never saw her there again, so God had really just sent her there for me. As soon I started taking probiotics, the bloating stopped, and I still take them with my supplements.

Towards the end of 2018 my body was so run down from the stress at work and having to deal with the nursing and the loss of my mother earlier in 2018 that I got so sick again with a chest infection. I went to consult with my doctor and I found a locum male doctor again, who unfortunately was the opposite of the nice lady I had consulted with before. He actually did not examine me at all. He asked me for my symptoms and then gave me medication whilst he was supposed to give me a prescription. But you know, when you are not well sometimes either your mind just goes to sleep or you don't have the energy to question. He was rather very nice, though. He was very talkative and during our conversation he told me that he had been a top student in his matric year in the Eastern Cape and had gone to Tuba to study medicine but was now hating it. It was very sad for me to hear that especially as someone who conducts career guidance sessions in order to help people find their purpose so that they don't find themselves doing something they hate just for the sake of money.

It was on a Friday, so after the consultation I left the practice and rested for the whole weekend. I felt better and the next Monday I went back to work. When I was at work, I could not stop coughing to the extent that I had to go back to the doctor and this time, fortunately, I was attended to by the actual owner of the practice who is very good.

On this day, what was interesting was that I had to be the good Samaritan. When my time came for my consultation the doctor was nowhere to be found. He had snuck out as if he was going out quickly to return in no time. Myself and other patients waited and, for some reason, I decided to be calm. Something told me that something must have happened. The doctor eventually came back and it was my turn. Just as I entered his consulting room he started by saying 'I'm sorry mam, please forgive me but can I just

The beautiful thing with having an intimate relationship with God is that He leads you in ways you would have never imagined.

vent? People forget that doctors are also human beings. I had to rush home to attend to my wife who is on insulin and because of load shedding we have not been able to charge her syringe for her medication and the meat at home has gone bad since the fridges have been off. I then had to go and fetch my kids from school. In addition I have not slept and I had not bathed earlier because my friend's daughter, who is a doctor, who is out of the country had to be admitted to hospital for an operation and I had to facilitate all of that'.

I sat in front of this doctor, with my own chest discomfort and coughing, and just listened. Then I extended my condolences to him and assured him that I got him and that I was sorry that the patients were being so insensitive towards him. He then eventually attended to me and examined me properly and told me that my sinuses were swollen and that I needed to take a whole week off as I was worn out from stress. He also gave me a vitamin B injection and antibiotics and told me I needed to look after myself. He said this with a very stern face. I went home and really rested that week. The following week I had recuperated sufficiently and was back at work.

Within the same year in this job I think - due to a lot of stress - even my hair started thinning, my nails were breaking and were not growing. I tried to take hair and nail supplements, but they were not helping. At the beginning of 2019 my body started itching very badly and I started feeling fatigued constantly. I consulted different doctors about the itching and all they would give me were antibiotics and cortisone which would stop the itching temporarily. The itching was so bad that it was affecting my sleep and my appetite. I started losing weight.

Eventually, I went to see a specialist for allergy tests and all of them were negative. This specialist asked me to do some blood tests and the results showed that my white blood cells count was very low. Then I realised I had to confront the giant of ARVs again as it had become apparent that my immune system was now very weak. Then I shared with my prayer partner about my status and about what I had been going through. She responded with so much compassion and said she never would have thought since I looked so healthy and always carried myself with so much courage.

During this time I was also invited to speak at a women's conference and the Holy Spirit led me to share my testimony. The exact Words the Holy Spirit said to me were: "There is going to be at least one person who is going to be delivered from your testimony." Indeed there was one lady who came up to me after the conference and shared that she was in such a state of confusion as she had just been diagnosed with the virus. She was so thankful that I had shared as she was encouraged.

Before I went to the conference I shared with my prayer partner what the Holy Spirit had said to me. I needed someone to keep me accountable so that I didn't withdraw. She assured me that she would be praying with me. I have never doubted that God would heal me completely but I also allowed God to take me through the process of learning to trust Him and to wait on Him. It has also become very clear to me that my life is not my own and it is for God to use it to reach others who are going through pain and so I have learned to trust my Daddy and be obedient because He is all knowing after all and His promises are 'Yes' and 'Amen'. He has promised that He will turn my mourning into dancing.

"You turned my wailing into dancing; you removed my sackcloth and clothed me with joy, that my heart may sing your praises and not be silent. Lord my God I will praise you forever." (Psalm 30:11-12 NIV)

"For his anger lasts only a moment, but his favour lasts a lifetime; weeping may stay for the night, but rejoicing comes in the morning." (Psalm 30"5 NIV)

Since the itching was becoming really bad, and was affecting my sleep as well as my appetite, I then consulted with my doctor who had not known my status before. My doctor usually has a lot of locum doctors, some of whom have been really bad, but this time I was attended to by a retired elderly doctor who was very nice. After sharing my history with him he then shared a story with me of one of his patients who had consulted him because she wanted to start taking ARVs. He says he suggested that they do the test again as a standard procedure and the results came back negative. He says this patient broke down in tears when she discovered she had been healed because five years previously she had tested positive and she had never told anyone.

As this doctor was telling me the story I could just see God speaking through him and giving me hope that one day I would be completely healed. I just needed to hold on and trust Him. It was as if God was saying that no matter what was happening right now, if I trusted Him I would see the end. I was so encouraged. God used this doctor to encourage me yet again and to remain hopeful.

So we did an HIV test as a standard procedure. We also did tests for viral load, CD4 count, liver and kidneys. The results reflected the viral load as 29 000 (very high), the CD4 count as 40 (very low) and the liver and kidneys in perfect condition. By the way it is not very good when the viral load is high and the CD4 count is low, but then again God had preserved my life as a CD4 count of 40 qualifies as AIDS and all sorts of opportunistic diseases, but I had none of those. I told my doctor I was ready to try out ARVs again and I asked him if there were options other than the TRIBUSS that had made me sick before.

He suggested that we go speak to the main doctor. The main doctor made a comment that I looked very healthy and I didn't look like I had HIV. Little did these people know that every time someone made a positive statement about my health it made me hear God speaking right into my heart, giving me hope that one day I would be healed completely. You see, when you have experienced God's miraculous hand you cannot help but believe that He will do it again, so I keep on believing for a miracle because I know that all things are possible with Him and to those that believe. Sometimes in the midst of pain and uncertainty you just need to hear a Word of encouragement from God while waiting for a breakthrough.

The main doctor also acknowledged that they have had reports of issues with bad side effects from previous ARVs but – that said - there were new ARVs which were now proving to be better and he suggested one of the recent drugs called the Agriptega. We filled in forms so they could put me on a chronic programme with my medical aid. All was approved except my medical aid said there would be a co-payment for Agriptega as it is very expensive. I agreed and started taking the medication.

My body responded very badly to it. My skin started breaking out and the itching started becoming worse. I went back to my doctor and he gave me antibiotics as well as some creams but these did not help. A month later I went back to him and told him to change the medication. We changed the ARVs to Trivenz and my body responded well except the itching still continued. I then noticed that some of the foods I was eating were triggering it so I started eliminating most foods and became a vegan until I saw a dermatologist who explained that it's a common reaction for people who are HIV positive and who have just starting to take ARVs. It's usually a good sign that the body is responding faster to the medication and since the immune system is picking up so fast it is bringing other ailments to the surface which could have been lying dormant.

She gave me cortisone and some tablets to manage the itching until the ARVs settled into my body. So here's the thing. We have been told so many times that people should not stop taking their ARVs otherwise the body will be resistant to them the next time. My argument here is that what people miss saying is that maybe if the person tries to take the same kind of drug the body might become resistant to them if they tried to take them again, however there are different kinds of ARVs which do leave room for someone to stop if they really have to. I speak from experience. I do understand that some things have been scientifically proven, but the reality is there are some experiences that go against science especially when it comes to spiritual matters. After all, God is the greatest and miraculous scientist who does things that sometimes do not make sense.

66

"It's not the years in your life that counts, it's the life in your years"

– *Abe Lincoln*

CHAPTER 8
DEALING WITH RELATIONSHIPS

I must say that for most of life since I have embarked on my journey to fulfil destiny, relationships have never been a priority to me. After my experience with Max (the guy who suggested I go for the HIV test) and after my diagnosis I decided to remain single, partly because I could not imagine having to disclose my status and be rejected.

It is sad that there are people who deliberately get into relationships with the aim of infecting other people. This has never crossed my mind at all for various reasons. Firstly, I have always believed that God can heal HIV and He will heal me. Secondly, Jesus delivered me from being vindictive. I have always understood that I have one enemy in this world and it is the devil. Thirdly, I have always believed in taking responsibility for my actions. At some point in my life I was stupid and naïve and I made decisions that made me suffer the consequences of my own actions. I have also always believed that God loves His people so much that instead of inflicting pain on them He shows them His goodness so that they might repent. The Word of God commands me to 'Love my neighbour as myself' (Matthew 22:39; Mark 12:32). I have a responsibility as a child of God to love my neighbour as myself so that God can be glorified through my life.

In many instances I have been happy that some men ended up pursuing me instead of others who could have deliberately infected them. I have had plenty of opportunities to infect others but I made sure I protected those people because I love them, I fear God and mostly because God loves them. I have two friends that infected their partners. I cannot even explain what was going on in their minds and I don't judge them because it was back in the days when HIV was still a taboo subject. Both of them had been faithful in their relationships when they contracted the virus but they suffered because of the unfaithfulness of their partners. They both went through hell during those times and I don't think I even did enough to try and put myself in their shoes. Sometimes I thought they were dramatic but all I did was stick by their side and allowed them to be.

As mentioned earlier, I made a decision to live and not focus so much on my HIV status. So, at some point I opened my heart to relationships. I met a very handsome man – I'll call him Xola. Someone's looks is not what primarily determines getting into a relationship with someone but Xola charmed me with his handsome looks and his big beautiful eyes, so it was impossible to ignore him. Since I was always looking for a serious relationship I made a decision to disclose my status upfront before I got serious with anyone. I liked Xola a lot and we had a very special connection. So I disclosed my status.

The next day he was nowhere to be found and I concluded that he had run away. A few years later he came back and confessed that my disclosure was not the reason he ran away, but that he had been laid off at work and was ashamed and could not face me, so he left the province altogether and by that time I had moved on.

Then I met Bobo. He was such a gentleman and paid a lot of attention to detail. We also had a very special connection. I also told him about my status and he responded positively. He said he did not have a problem with it and assured me that he loved me no matter what and he actually told me he wanted to marry me. He had met my family, my Pastors, my friends and was very serious about making me his wife.

I later discovered that Bobo was 'semi-married', for a lack of a better word. He had been staying with someone for six years and she was pregnant with his second child. I also discovered that actually he had an older child from a different woman which he had not disclosed to me. My heart was so broken but I was so glad that God had revealed it before I got into the marriage. I quickly dealt with it and moved on with my life.

Then I met Thulani. Thulani was very charming, handsome and funny. He was also a visionary which was something that attracted me to him. His vision of making a difference in communities through education was very similar to mine. I disclosed my status to Thulani. He was fine with it and he stuck around. Then I discovered Thulani was in the process of finalising a divorce which I was uncomfortable with because I felt he was opening a door while another door had not been closed so I initially refused his proposal for a relationship. I later decided to give him a chance when I discovered he had not given up. Thulani has six children with six different women and for someone of his calibre and his age I really started to wonder why he had not been married. While in the process of finalising the relationship I discovered that he was very selfish, very self-centred and was living a lie based on experiences I had with him. I then decided to have nothing to do with him.

After several more failed relationships I decided to close the door for relationships. I thank God I have learned to channel my desire for intimacy to Him and I spend a lot of time in the presence of God. It is the most fulfilling thing a person can ever do. One thing I need to mention is that sometimes, in my previous relationships, although I had committed to keeping myself holy I would fall into sin. This was until, one day, I was watching a preaching by one man of God and he happened to talk about sexual sin. He said, 'Every time you sleep with someone you are engaging with the demons that person is carrying, for example if that person is carrying 17 demons, they sleep with you, they transfer their 17 demons onto you, then they go and sleep with someone else who has 24 demons, they come back and transfer those 24 demons onto and you end up with 41

"I know your works, that you are neither cold nor hot. I could wish you were cold or hot. So then because you are lukewarm, and neither cold nor hot, I will vomit out of My mouth."
(Revelation 3: 15-16)

demons, then you wonder why things are not going well in your life.'

The Holy Spirit later revealed to me that demons activate certain spirits. If you have a demon that is carrying a spirit of poverty, you will be poor; if you have a demon that is carrying a spirit of lust, you will be lustful and so forth. This was so scary to me to an extent that if the enemy tried to tempt me with sexual sin I would imagine demons being transferred to me and I would literally run. In fact, I have since refrained from putting myself in vulnerable positions such as being with a man I am attracted to in a private place.

More than anything I made a decision to become celibate because it is God's mandate for me as His child. God's judgement is real and I fear the consequences of sin. If God is faithful in performing His Word of blessings, surely He is faithful to His Word of punishing sin as merciful and gracious as He is. So many times we have misused the mercy and grace of God and He is tired of it. As children of God we cannot live a double life otherwise we will be exposed. I hope and pray that children of God will not engage in sexual activities outside of marriage. I know what it is like to suffer the consequences of sin and I do not wish it for anybody else. That is why I am writing this book. As a child of God run from sexual sin as much as you can; it's for your own good.

"I know your works, that you are neither cold nor hot. I could wish you were cold or hot. So then because you are lukewarm, and neither cold nor hot, I will vomit out of My mouth." (Revelation 3: 15-16)

In verse 19, Jesus continues and says "As many as I love, I rebuke and chasten. Therefore be zealous and repent."

It is very clear here that Jesus does not condemn us when we fall into sin, and please note that there is a difference between 'swimming in sin' and 'falling into sin'. Someone who is swimming in sin is usually the one who is lukewarm and, even in this state, Jesus urges you to repent (change your ways, stop sinning) but if it happens that you refuse to repent, He will vomit you or expose you to what is happening to many believers in our days. It is possible to live a life that sin free because of God's grace.

"For the grace of God has appeared that offers salvation to all people. It teaches us to say 'No' to ungodliness and worldly passions, and to live self-

controlled, upright and godly lives in the present age while we wait for the blessed hope, the appearing of the glory of our great God and Saviour, Jesus Christ, who gave himself for us to redeem us from all wickedness and to purity for himself a people that are his very own, eager to do what is good."

One day I had a conversation with the Holy Spirit and He asked me: 'Which void are you trying to fill?' I was forced to do some introspection and ask myself what it was I was really looking for. I realised that the void I was trying to fill only God could fill.

I then made a decision to fall in love with my Father, give Him my heart fully and to follow His principles regarding marriage.

I'm sure by now you are shaking your head, but the reality is that human beings were crated for love and for touch. No matter how much we can lie to ourselves - especially if we have been through hurtful relationships - we cannot change that we all long to be loved and nobody wants to die alone, at least I don't. But you see I believe women have been empowered to be successful and confident as well as to be strong for everyone else, but women have not been taught to be vulnerable. I have learned that vulnerability is actually the greatest strength a woman can ever have. That is why I am writing this book. I have learned to be so vulnerable that I want to help other women to allow themselves to be so that they can confront their giants truthfully and effectively. So many women wear masks and try very hard to be who they are not because they are afraid of being judged by society.

I write this book to break this stronghold and to be a voice that encourages you to be honest about how you feel and be free to talk about it. Be honest about your anger, disappointments, loneliness and about your fears of not being sure if you will ever meet the right person. Be honest about the fact that sometimes you have nightmares of someone mistreating and abusing you. Men also have their own fears. I'm not a man but from what I have seen men have been pushed to the back by society so many times they are scared to take up their places of leadership and caring for their loved ones in case they appear to be controlling.

Men also probably have fears of marrying women who will end up being the man of the house in wanting to make decisions so that the man has no voice. Men also have fears that they will marry a woman who will mistake their vulnerability for weakness. A lot of men have grown up without fathers and I don't care how society can justify single parenting, it is abnormal. No child was meant to grow up without a father especially a boy child. Fathers have a masculinity they carry which they transfer onto their sons. If a man has never had a father in their lives they tend to experience a void that might result in them being vulnerable in many areas of their lives.

Some men treat women based on what they see in society or based on their own intuition and then later realise how abusive they are. These thoughts might then haunt them while they are going through a process of restoration. It is during this process that they will need their women as being the ear and the comfort as well as the assurance that it is all going to be OK.

Besides the fact that I decided to be celibate, I decided I would not get into a relationship until I had followed certain principles:

- Marriage is for advancing the Kingdom of God.
- I cannot be unequally yoked, which means whoever I marry must be born again.
- A real man must pursue me. Men are hunters and they were created like that. "He who finds a wife finds a good thing, and obtains favour from the Lord." (Proverbs 18:22).
- I am called to be a suitable helper to someone I am comparable to (Genesis 2:18). After creating Adam God gave him a command to 'till the ground' then He gave him a 'helper'. I cannot help anyone if they do not have a vision in life.
- Marriage is a platform for me to thrive in fulfilling my purpose in life.

"

"One of the ways to fight stigma and empower HIV-positive people is by speaking out openly and honestly about who we are and what we experience"

– Alex Garner - HIV Activist

CHAPTER 9
CONSIDERING IT JOY

"Consider it pure joy, my brothers and sisters, whenever you face trials of many kinds, because you know that the testing of your faith produces perseverance. Let perseverance finish its work so that you may be mature and complete, not lacking anything" (James 1:2-3 NIV)

At some point I reflected upon my life and with all the hurdles I have had to cross I wondered how I made it. The Holy Spirit said to me: "You have managed to protect your faith." This made me realise that in every trying situations our faith is always being tested and if it is genuine, it will pass, but if not it will fail. My HIV journey has also helped me to understand the book of Job better which many people misinterpret. I was diagnosed with HIV at a point in my life when I had given up everything to follow God. I was living out my purpose and serving God faithfully and so at some point I didn't understand how God could reward me with this painful journey. As I read the book of Job over and over again I got to understand my own journey.

"There was a man in the land of Uz, whose name was Job; and that man was blameless and upright, and one who feared God and shunned evil." (Job 1:1 NKJV)

Point 1: Job was blameless, feared God and shunned evil.

"Now there was a day when the sons of God came to present themselves before the Lord, and Satan also came among them. And the Lord said to Satan, 'From where do you come?' So Satan answered the Lord and said, 'From going to and from on the earth, and from walking back and forth on it.' Then the Lord said to Satan, 'Have you considered My servant Job, that there is none like him on the earth, a blameless and upright man, one who fears God and shuns evil?'"(Job 1: 6-8 NKJV)

Point 2: God is one who suggested Job for consideration by Satan.

"So Satan answered the Lord and said, 'Does Job fear God for nothing? Have you not made a hedge around him, around his household, and around all that he has on every side? You have blessed the work of his hands, and his possessions have increased in the land. But now, stretch our Your hand and touch all that he has, and he will surely curse You to Your face!'" (Job 1:9-11 NKJV)

Point 3: Satan knew that Job feared God. Satan also knew that God had protected Job and that he could not have access to Job nor to anything he owned.

Point 4: Satan's plan is so that we could curse God to His face because He knows, without God, we are nothing.

"And the Lord said to Satan, 'Behold, all that he has is in your power; only do not lay a hand on his person.'" (Job 1: 12 NKJV)

Point 5: God gave Satan permission to destroy all that Job had.

"In all this Job did not sin nor charge God with wrong." (Job 1:22 NKJV)

Point 6: Job remained faithful to God because He knew that God is a good God. He would not of His own want to destroy Job. God also knew that Job was so faithful and committed to Him that He would not curse Him to His face no matter what. And Job indeed passed the test.

I would encourage you to read the whole book of Job in order to understand the entire context. I pray that it will bless you just as much as it blessed me and helped me to stay on course in the midst of my HIV challenges.

I have seen many people turn their backs on God when they have gone through suffering in their lives. And so, as I conclude, I hope my testimony will encourage you to hold on to God as He is not a man that He should lie nor a Son that He should change His mind.

I am secure in my relationship with my Daddy God right now and nothing, and no pain, will ever make me turn my back on Him. The last time I checked, my HIV status was still positive, but I continue to trust Him for complete healing because of the following scriptures:

"And Jesus went about all Galilee, teaching in their synagogues, and preaching the gospel of the kingdom, and healing all manner of sickness and all manner of disease among the people." (Matthew 4:23 KJV)

"And Jesus went about all the cities and villages, teaching in their synagogues, and preaching the gospel of the kingdom, and healing every sickness and every disease among the people." (Matthew 9:35 KJV)

"As Jesus was on his way, the crowds almost crushed him. And the woman was there who had been subject to bleeding for twelve years, but no one could heal her. She came up behind him and touched the edge of his cloak, and immediately her bleeding stopped." (Luke 8: 42-44 NIV)

"...being fully confident of this, that he who began a good work in you will carry it on to completion until the day of Jesus Christ." (Philippians 1:6 NIV)

"The thief comes only to steal and kill and destroy; I have come that they may have life, and have it to the full" (John 10:10 NIV)

"But he was pierced for our transgressions, he was crushed for our iniquities; the punishment that brought us peace was on him, and by his wounds we are healed." (Isaiah 53:5 NIV)

"In the midst of challenges, it's very important to guard your faith because without faith it is impossible to please God." (Hebrews 11:6)

So, play through the pain (Late Dr Myles Munroe) knowing that...

"The end of the matter is better than its beginning." (Ecclesiastes 7:8)

"

---

*"Education, prevention
and awareness are key, but
stigmatization and exclusion
from family is what makes
people suffer most"*

– Ralph Fiennes

APPENDIX

Let me clarify that ARVs DO NOT CURE HIV. They simply reduce the viral load in the body making the virus inactive. When the virus is 'undetected' it means chances of infecting someone with the virus are very slim.

It is therefore important that when someone is taking ARVs:

1. They eat well
2. They take supplements
3 They drink lots of water (at least two litres a day)
4. They exercise (while the immune system is still weak walks also make a difference)

In 2003, years before I was diagnosed with the virus, I had minor ailments and was also struggling with my weight so I decided to start eating healthy. A friend of mine was listening to the radio and she heard Mary-Ann Shearer share her testimony and about her book called 'Living healthy the natural way'. She recommended this book to me and because I was so desperate I bought the book, read it in one day and applied its principles. Some of the principles that Mary-Ann emphasises in the book are:

1. That our bodies were designed to survive on natural foods.
2. Our bodies talk to us and therefore we must listen to our bodies.
3. The combinations of the foods we eat will determine the health of our bodies.
4. Because we all have different genes your body might respond well to some foods.
5. Meat is a cause of most ailments in the body.

After reading the book I decided to eat a lot of fruit and vegetables and I automatically lost my taste for meat and most junk foods. For five years I was a vegan[1].

Before following the principles in the book I used to suffer from bad hay fever and had been on chronic medication for years. I also struggled with fatigue and other minor ailments. Within that five years of being a vegan I was completely healed from hay fever and I stopped taking the medication. My energy and my skin improved and my health in general improved tremendously. I lost a lot of weight and I never had to go on diets again.

Here are some of the natural foods that my body has responded well to:

Future Life (Although processed it's usually good for breakfast)

Fruit (Paw Paw, Oranges, Strawberries). Fruit need to be combined appropriately otherwise they can cause indigestion. Avoid mixing citrus fruits with sugar fruits, for example oranges and bananas.

---

1   A person who does not eat or use animal products

Nectarines
Plums
Peaches
Cucumber
Lettuce
Tomatoes (Has sometimes been a bit acidic for my body so I don't eat much of them)
Avocadoes
Lentils
Butternut
Carrots
Broccoli
Green Beans
Sugar beans
Beetroot
Sweet potatoes
Potatoes
Peppers
Mushrooms
Onions
Spinach

Important to note is that I avoid spices as much as I can. I also avoid soups and stocks as they tend to have spices. I cook my food with salt, paprika (exception), mixed herbs, thyme, garlic, parsley.

Supplements

I usually change my supplements every three months so that my body does not become resistant to them. Changing the brands might also help.

Month 1-3
Viral Guard (Has probiotic)
Slow mag (Mornings)
Calcium (Evenings, also helps with sleeping)

Month 3-6
Immunice
Probiotics (Helps with indigestion and bloating)
Calcium and Magnesium combined (NGC product)

Additional
Zinc (Listen to your body, sometimes my body does not like it – so I take it once in a while)
Folic Acid
Acc 200 (For flu symptoms)
Vitamin C
Vitamin D
Multivitamins (Any brand that works for you, the more expensive brands are usually effective)

RECIPES

I have included 3 easy recipes for 3 of my favourite meals. These are easy to make and are healthy and nutritious. Enjoy!

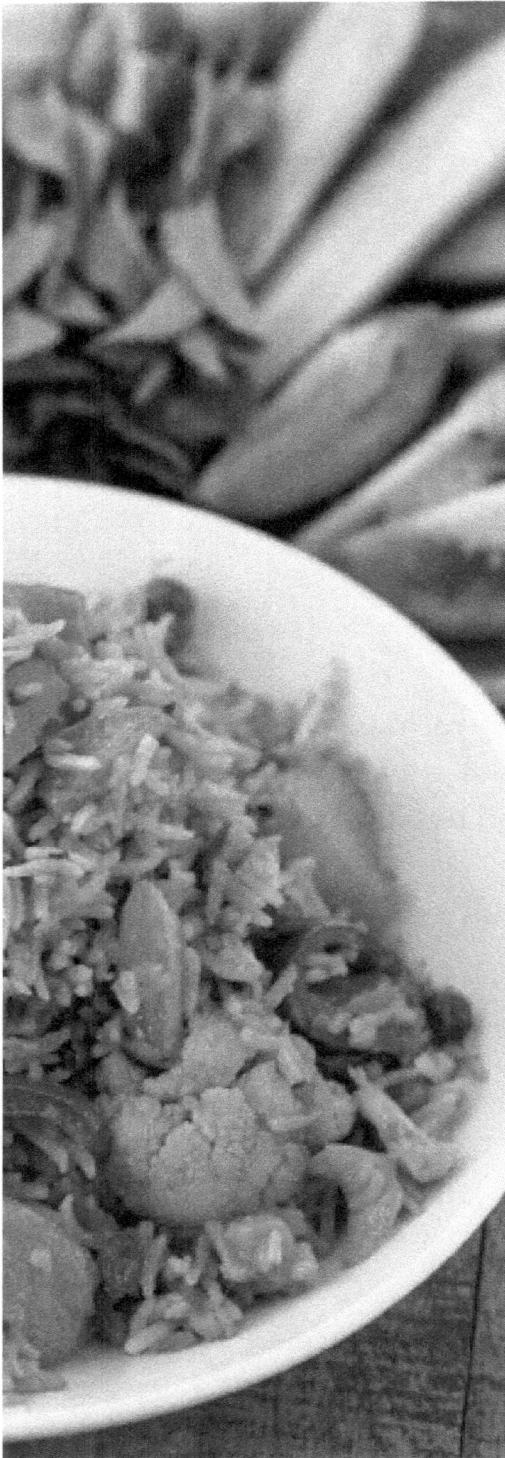

MEAL 1
VEGETABLE BIRYANI

INGREDIENTS

Rice
Lentils
Onion
Peppers (Green/Yellow/Red)
Mushrooms
Olive Oil
Salt
Paprika
Mixed Italian Herbs

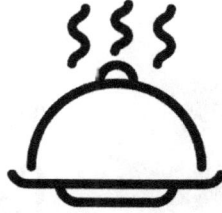

PROCESS

Step 1
Fry Onion and Green pepper in olive oil, once cooked add mushrooms, salt, paprika and mixed/italian herbs.

Step 2
Boil rice until cooked

Step 3
Boil lentils until cooked (they cook very quickly, make sure they are not mushy)

Step 4
Mix everything together and serve

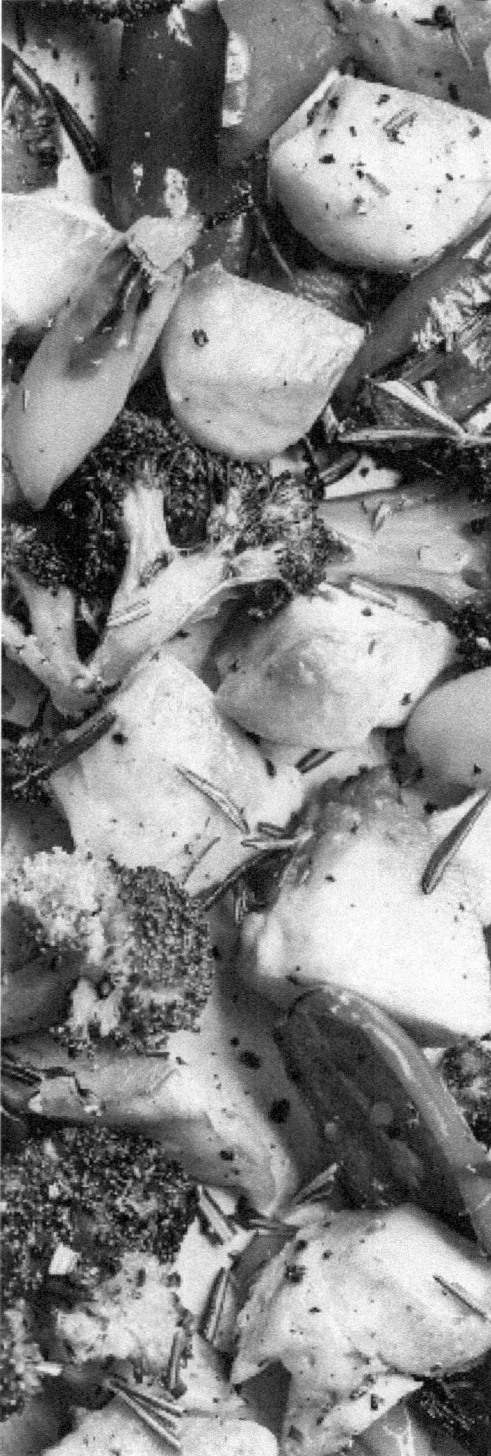

MEAL 2
CHICKEN BREASTS AND VEGETABLES

INGREDIENTS

Chicken breast – 1 or 2 trays
Onion
Peppers (Green, Yellow and Red – you don't have to use all of them, whatever you prefer)
Salt
Mixed/Italian herbs
Paprika
Broccoli
Olive Oil
Carrots
Beetroot
Bisto gravy

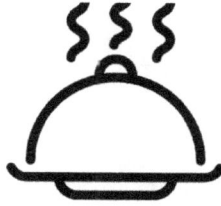

PROCESS

Step 1
Boil Beetroot until soft – grate it and add chutney
(ready to serve-sometimes I eat it alone)

Step 2
Cut chicken breasts into small pieces – add salt, mixed herbs,
paprika and mix together, add onion and pepper/s then add olive boil.
Bring to the stove to fry.

Step 3
Mix 1 to 2 spoons of Bisto soup with cold water – half a cup of water

Step 4
Add Bisto soup to chick breast mixture once soft. If the
soup is too thick, you can always add more water.

Step 5
Make sure the fire is low, let it boil until ready.

Step 6
Cut up carrots in slices, add a bit of salt, sugar, mixed herbs, paprika,
olive oil . Mix together and bring to the stove to fry until cooked – (Some
people like their carrots soft and some like it crispy – your choice)

Step 7
Cut up Broccoli and wash thoroughly – add very little water and bring to
the stove, once cooked add a bit of salt and olive oil (it cooks very quickly)

Step 8
Once everything is cooked – Serve

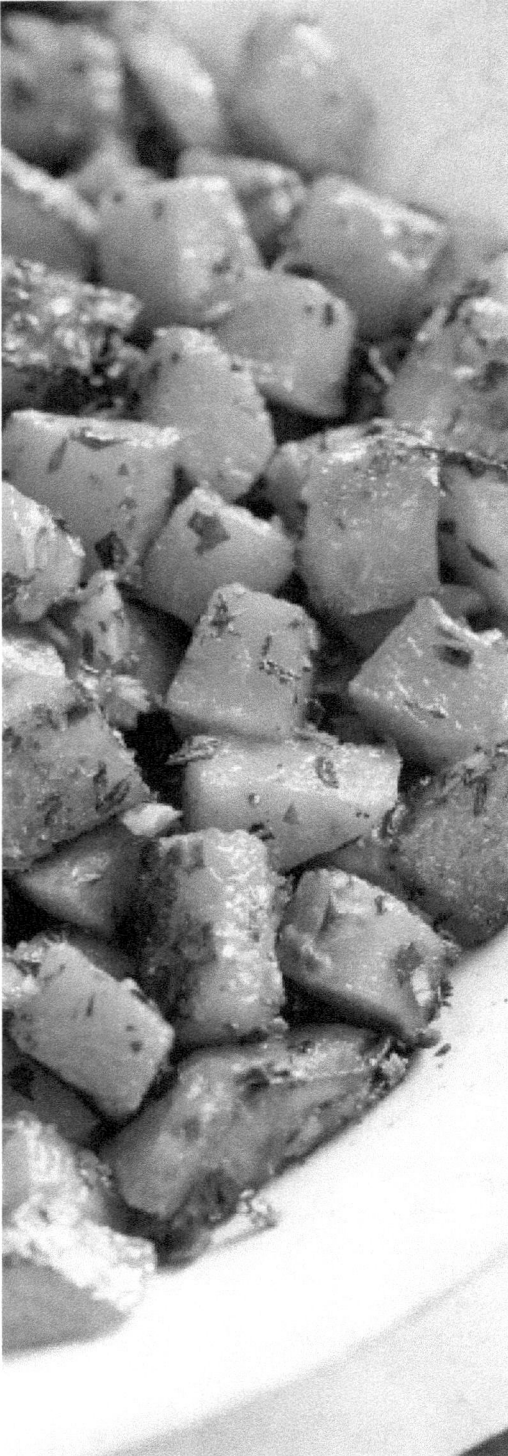

MEAL 3
PLAIN
VEGETARIAN

INGREDIENTS

Butternut
Lentils
Sweet potatoes/Potatoes
Onion
Peppers (Green/yelllo/Red)
Mushrooms
Bisto Gravy
Salt
Paprika
Mixed/Italian Herbs
Greek salad (Lettuce,
cucumber, tomatoe, feta,
olives,peppers avocado)

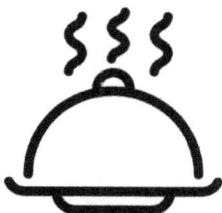

PROCESS

Step 1
Cut out potatoes/sweet potatoes into wedges

Step 2
Boil potatoes briefly add salt, bask them in olive oil

Step 3
Bake in oven

Step 4
Cook other butternut as you wish

Step 5
Fry Onion, Peppers in olive oil add salt, mixed and
paprika – once cooked add mushrooms and bisto gravy.

Step 6
Cut out salad ingredients into small pieces including lettuce –
they usually look edible and are easy to eat if they are cut in small pieces.

Step 7
Serve

www.ingramcontent.com/pod-product-compliance
Lightning Source LLC
Chambersburg PA
CBHW021337290326
41933CB00038B/884